P9-DTF-727

CONCISE GUIDE TO

Mood Disorders

RENEWALS 458-4574

M.

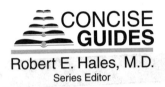

CONCISE GUIDES

Robert E. Hales, M.D.
Series Editor

CONCISE GUIDE TO
Mood Disorders

Steven L. Dubovsky, M.D.

Professor of Psychiatry and Medicine
Vice Chair, Department of Psychiatry
Departments of Psychiatry and Medicine
University of Colorado School of Medicine
Denver, Colorado

Amelia N. Dubovsky, B.A.

Graduate Studies
Columbia University
New York, New York

WITHDRAWN
UTSA Libraries

American
Psychiatric
Publishing, Inc.

Washington, DC
London, England

Note: The authors have worked to ensure that all information in this book is accurate at the time of publication and consistent with general psychiatric and medical standards, and that information concerning drug dosages, schedules, and routes of administration is accurate at the time of publication and consistent with standards set by the U.S. Food and Drug Administration and the general medical community. As medical research and practice continue to advance, however, therapeutic standards may change. Moreover, specific situations may require a specific therapeutic response not included in this book. For these reasons and because human and mechanical errors sometimes occur, we recommend that readers follow the advice of physicians directly involved in their care or the care of a member of their family.

Books published by American Psychiatric Publishing, Inc., represent the views and opinions of the individual authors and do not necessarily represent the policies and opinions of APPI or the American Psychiatric Association.

Copyright © 2002 American Psychiatric Publishing, Inc.
ALL RIGHTS RESERVED

DSM-IV-TR criteria are reprinted from American Psychiatric Association: *Diagnostic and Statistical Manual of Mental Disorders,* 4th Edition, Text Revision. Washington, DC, American Psychiatric Association, 2000. Used with permission. Copyright 2000, American Psychiatric Association.

This Concise Guide was developed in part from Dubovsky SL, Davies R, Dubovsky A: "Mood Disorders," in *The American Psychiatric Publishing Textbook of Clinical Psychiatry,* Fourth Edition. Edited by Hales RE, Yudofsky SC. Washington, DC, American Psychiatric Publishing, 2003. Copyright 2003 American Psychiatric Publishing, Inc. Used with permission.

Manufactured in the United States of America on acid-free paper
06 05 04 03 02   5 4 3 2 1
First Edition

Typeset in Adobe's Times and Helvetica

American Psychiatric Publishing, Inc.
1400 K Street, N.W.
Washington, DC 20005
www.appi.org

Library of Congress Cataloging-in-Publication Data
Dubovsky, Steven L.
  Concise guide to mood disorders / Steven L. Dubovsky, Amelia N. Dubovsky.–1st ed.
    p. ; cm
  Includes bibliographical references and index.
  ISBN 1-58562-056-4 (alk. paper)
    1. Affective disorders. 2. Depression, Mental. I. Dubovsky, Amelia N., 1979– II. Title.
  [DNLM: 1. Mood Disorders. WM 171 D818c 2002]
RC537.D83 2002
616.85'27–dc21
                                                                    2002067897

British Library Cataloguing in Publication Data
A CIP record is available from the British Library.

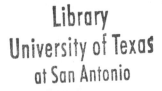

Library
University of Texas
at San Antonio

To Anne and Liz

CONTENTS

LIST OF TABLES

Introduction

1 Diagnosing Mood Disorders

4 Somatic Therapies for Mood Disorders

5 Psychotherapies for Mood Disorders

6 Integrated Treatment of Unipolar Depression

7 Integrated Treatment of Bipolar Disorder

LIST OF FIGURES

INTRODUCTION

to the Concise Guides Series

The Concise Guides Series from American Psychiatric Publishing, Inc., provides, in an accessible format, practical information for psychiatrists, psychiatry residents, and medical students working in a variety of treatment settings, such as inpatient psychiatry units, outpatient clinics, consultation-liaison services, and private office settings. The Concise Guides are meant to complement the more detailed information to be found in lengthier psychiatry texts.

The Concise Guides address topics of special concern to psychiatrists in clinical practice. The books in this series contain a detailed table of contents, along with an index, tables, figures, and other charts for easy access. The books are designed to fit into a lab coat pocket or jacket pocket, which makes them a convenient source of information. References have been limited to those most relevant to the material presented.

Robert E. Hales, M.D., M.B.A.
Series Editor, American Psychiatric Publishing Concise Guides

PREFACE

The exploding body of information about mood disorders presents important opportunities for clinicians treating these common problems, but it may also seem overwhelming at times. This book is a condensed yet comprehensive overview of current knowledge about the pathophysiology, psychology, and treatment of mood disorders. First, we briefly review the epidemiology of mood disorders. We then discuss complexities of diagnosis and explain how dimensional aspects of diagnosis add to the traditional categorical diagnoses. Etiologies of mood disorders are addressed next. Finally, somatic and psychosocial therapies and likely outcomes of treatment are discussed at length.

A challenge in any concise guide is to distill complicated information in a manner that makes essential concepts easily accessible. This is particularly important in a discussion of mood disorders. New ideas about diagnosis of mood disorders have the potential to transform traditional approaches to understanding mood disorders and planning treatment. New concepts in cell and molecular biology have led to an increased understanding of the progression of other medical illnesses. These concepts have the potential to elucidate why mood disorders become more complex and treatment resistant over time, and to inform development of more effective and precise therapies.

We have limited the number of references cited to essential reviews and studies; a complete summary of the medical literature would have taken up the entire book. Readers interested in a more comprehensive reference list can obtain one from us. We are hopeful that this concise summary will prove useful to anyone dealing with mood disorders in the real world who does not have time for an extensive review of research data.

INTRODUCTION

I am tired of tears and laughter,
And men that laugh and weep;
Of what may come hereafter
For men that sow and reap:
I am weary of days and hours,
Blown buds of barren flowers,
Desires and dreams and powers
And everything but sleep.

—*Algernon Charles Swinburne*

Mood disorders are among the most common medical disorders. Although many clinicians are familiar with the obvious forms of depression and mania, more subtle and complex forms are more difficult to recognize. In this book, we present a condensed but comprehensive approach to the diagnosis and treatment of all mood disorders.

■ EPIDEMIOLOGY

In the United States, the lifetime risk of a major depressive episode is estimated to be around 6%, and the lifetime risk of any mood disorder is said to be around 8% (Cassem 1995). The point prevalence of major depression ranges from 2.6% to 5.5% among men and from 6.0% to 11.8% among women (Kessler et al. 1994). The prevalence of dysthymia is 3%–4% (Keller et al. 1996). Some reports suggest that as many as 48% of Americans have had one or more affective episodes (Cassem 1995). Most studies have found unipolar depression (major depressive disorder and dysthymia) to be twice as common in women as in men (Kessler et al. 1994). The meaning of the sex difference, which is not apparent until adolescence, remains to be clarified but probably involves differences in role strain as much as hormonal effects. Sex does not appear to affect the prevalence of bipolar disorder. The prevalence of major depression in primary care practice is 4.8%–9.2%, and the prevalence of all depressive disorders in primary care is 9%–20%, which makes mood disorders the most common psychiatric problems in primary care (McDaniel et al. 1995) and factors that increase the use of general health services (Weissman et al. 1988).

The effects of culture and social stress on the prevalence of depression were illustrated by a Cross-National Collaborative Group study, which used the Diagnostic Interview Schedule to make DSM-III (American Psychiatric Association 1980) diagnoses (Weissman et al. 1996). In this study involving 10 countries, the lifetime rate of major depression varied from a low of 1.5 cases per 100 adults in Taiwan to a high of 19.0 cases per 100 adults in Beirut, and the annual rate of depression was as low as 0.8 cases per 100 in Taiwan and as high as 5.8 per 100 in New Zealand. The importance of loss is illustrated by findings that the incidence of major depression is higher among separated or divorced people than among married individuals, especially men, and among medically ill patients (Lehtinen and Joukamaa 1994).

The prevalence of bipolar disorder is generally reported as being between 1% and 2.5%; however, some studies suggest rates for bipolar mood disorders of 3%–6.5% (Akiskal 1995). The frequency with which bipolar disorder is diagnosed probably depends on how it is defined, with broader definitions producing significantly higher rates (Akiskal 1995). Most prevalence studies require the presence of mania for a bipolar diagnosis to be recorded, but the bipolar II variant, which is characterized by episodes of hypomania but not mania, is more common than the bipolar I variant (Simpson et al. 1993). If mixed states and subsyndromal and complex forms of bipolar disorder are also considered (Akiskal 1995), the incidence of bipolar mood disorder is substantially higher.

When conservative criteria are used, at least 5%–15% of cases of adult depression are found to be bipolar (Bebbington 1995). On the other hand, Akiskal's group (Cassano et al. 1989) found that one-third of patients with primary depression met their criteria for bipolar spectrum disorders. The risk of bipolarity is higher among juveniles with major depression—at least 20% among depressed adolescents and 32% among depressed children younger than 11 years (Geller et al. 1996). In contrast to unipolar depression, the lifetime rate of classically defined bipolar disorder is relatively consistent across cultures, ranging from 0.3 cases per 100 individuals in Taiwan to 1.5 per 100 in New Zealand (Weissman et al. 1996).

In all industrialized countries of the world, the incidence of depression, mania, suicide, and psychotic mood disorders has been increasing in every generation since 1910 (Cross-National Collaborative Group 1992). There was an abrupt jump in the rate of increase for people born after 1940—a true increase in the incidence of mood disorders in subsequent generations (cohort effect), not a function of better recognition or more help-seeking (Cross-National Collaborative Group 1992). Not only are mood disorders becoming more common; they are also appearing at an earlier age (especially bipolar mood disorders). These changes seem to be due in part to anticipation, the accumulation of genetic risk across generations.

In worldwide surveys, depression is the fourth most important cause of disability and the fourth most costly medical illness. Depressed patients spend more time in bed than patients with diabetes, hypertension, arthritis, or chronic lung disease, and patients with depression have as much functional disability as patients with heart disease. Primary care physicians spend more time treating depression than treating hypertension, arteriosclerotic heart disease, or diabetes mellitus.

Suicide is an obvious public health problem that complicates mood disorders more frequently than other conditions. The lifetime risk of suicide among individuals with mood disorders is 10%–15% (Mueller and Leon 1996), and the risk of attempted suicide was increased 41-fold among depressed patients compared with those with other diagnoses, in the Epidemiologic Catchment Area surveys (Petronis et al. 1990). Women attempt suicide more frequently than men, but men are more likely to succeed. In one study, the excess risk of completed suicide among men was entirely accounted for by the higher prevalence of substance abuse among men and the greater likelihood that women have primary responsibility for children younger than 18 years (Young et al. 1994). The risk of suicide is high among people with mania as well as among those with depression. Patients with mixed bipolar states characterized by a combination of depression, rage, and grandiosity may be more likely to involve others in a suicide attempt—for example, through gunfights with the police. As many as 4% of people who commit suicide murder someone else first. High levels of distress and hopelessness increase the risk of suicide attempts among adolescents. Neuropsychological deficits are more common in depressed patients who have made high-lethality suicide attempts than in those who have made low-lethality attempts and in nonpatients, suggesting that impaired executive function may exist in people at risk for severe suicide attempts (Keilp et al. 2001).

Although many clinicians agree on factors that increase the risk of suicide, formal attempts to predict suicide have been disappointing. Suicide is such a rare event (about 11 per 100,000 deaths in the United States) that a prohibitively large number of patients would have to be followed prospectively to demonstrate that a constellation of features predicted an increased risk. In addition, no consensus exists concerning how long to follow a depressed patient before a conclusion can be made that suicide will not occur. There may be a statistically significant association between suicide and traditional risk factors such as older age, recent loss, male sex, bipolar depression, psychosis, comorbid substance abuse, history of a suicide attempt (especially if it was dangerous), and family history of suicide, but this association is not necessarily helpful in predicting suicide in an individual patient.

Despite the demonstrated inability of mental health professionals to predict (or prevent) suicide in a systematic manner, patients, families, and courts expect them to be able to do so. In an evaluation of immediate suicide risk, factors summarized in Table 1 can be

---

TABLE 1. **Factors suggesting an increased risk of suicide**

Demographic factors

Male sex

Recent loss

Never married

Older age

Symptoms

Severe depression

Anxiety

Hopelessness

Bipolar disorder

Psychosis, especially with command hallucinations

Current substance use

History

History of suicide attempts, especially if multiple or severe attempts

Family history of suicide

Suicidal thinking

Presence of a specific plan

Means available to carry out the plan

Absence of factors that would keep the patient from completing the plan

Rehearsal of the plan

---

considered. However, these factors at best suggest increased immediate risk. In addition, the short-term risk tends to fluctuate, and it is not known whether one risk factor is more important than another or how risk factors interact with each other. Given the current state of knowledge, it is probably impossible for anyone to predict with any accuracy the long-term risk of completed suicide.

Difficulty predicting suicide in the long run does not absolve clinicians from applying accumulated clinical wisdom to the management of the potentially suicidal patient. Because the majority of suicides occur in patients with psychiatric disorders, every psychiatric patient should be asked about suicide. One protocol for asking about suicide is presented in Table 2.

When a patient reports active thoughts of suicide, has a plan that could be carried out, and lacks credible factors that would pre-

TABLE 2. **Questions to ask the suicidal patient**

Have you felt bad enough to think about suicide?
What thoughts have you had?
Do you have a specific plan?
What is the plan?
Do you have the means to carry out the plan?
How close have you come to acting on it?
What has prevented you from acting on your thoughts?
Have you rehearsed the plan or made a secret attempt?

vent him or her from making an attempt, immediate steps must be taken to protect the patient. This is usually achieved through hospitalization, although in some cases the patient may remain at home or in a partial care setting under close observation. Although patients may be chronically suicidal for years, the acute risk of suicide usually does not last more than hours or days. While the patient is protected, steps can be taken to resolve the crisis that precipitated suicidality, reduce hopelessness, and institute treatment for depression. Most clinicians try to get patients to agree to "no suicide" contracts, but these have not been shown to be reliable. Patients who seem to feel better immediately after hospitalization may be concealing an active plan in order to be released and should be watched closely. In some cases, involuntary hospitalization may be necessary; in these situations, the likelihood of a lawsuit being successful is very low if the patient is later determined not to have been suicidal. On the other hand, a significant number of successful lawsuits in psychiatry concern patients who committed suicide shortly after having been allowed to refuse hospitalization or leave the hospital.

■ ECONOMICS OF MOOD DISORDERS

Depression produces more impairment of physical functioning, role functioning, social functioning, and perceived current health; is associated with more bodily pain; and causes patients to spend more days in bed because of poor health than does hypertension, diabetes, arthritis, or chronic pulmonary disease. In a study involving general medical patients in a health maintenance organization, patients with depressed mood or anhedonia of 2 weeks' duration but with an insufficient number of additional symptoms to meet full criteria for major depressive disorder still had 7.7 times as much impairment of social, family, and work functioning as patients without any depressive symptoms (Olfson 1996). The estimated total cost of depressive disorders in the United States was $44 billion in 1993 (Hall and Wise 1995). This is equivalent to the total cost of coronary heart disease, a condition that is no more prevalent and less readily treatable than depression. The direct costs of treating depression are about $12 billion, only $890 million of which is the cost of antidepressants (Hall and Wise 1995). Yet, third-party payers expend tremendous effort attempting to get physicians to prescribe cheaper antidepressants. The morbidity cost of depressive disorders in the United States is around $24 billion, and the mortality costs are $8 billion; these costs can be attributed in part to increased accident rates, substance abuse, development of somatic illnesses such as coronary heart disease, and increased use of medical hospitalization and outpatient treatment (Hall and Wise 1995).

■ REFERENCES

American Psychiatric Association: Diagnostic and Statistical Manual of Mental Disorders, 3rd Edition. Washington, DC, American Psychiatric Association, 1980

Akiskal HS: Le spectre bipolaire: acquisitions et perspectives cliniques. Encephale 21 (Spec No 6):3–11, 1995

Bebbington R: The epidemiology of bipolar affective disorder. Soc Psychiatry Psychiatr Epidemiol 30:279–292, 1995

Cassano GB, Akiskal HS, Musetti L, et al: Psychopathology, temperament, and past course in primary major depressions, 2: toward a redefinition of bipolarity with a new semistructured interview for depression. Psychopathology 22:278–288, 1989

Cassem EH: Depressive disorders in the medically ill: an overview. Psychosomatics 36:S2–S10, 1995

Cross-National Collaborative Group: The changing rate of major depression: cross-national comparisons. JAMA 268:3098–3105, 1992

Geller B, Todd RD, Luby J, et al: Treatment-resistant depression in children and adolescents. Psychiatr Clin North Am 19:253–265, 1996

Hall RC, Wise MG: The clinical and financial burden of mood disorders: cost and outcome. Psychosomatics 36:S11–S18, 1995

Keilp JG, Sackeim HA, Brodsky BS, et al: Neuropsychological dysfunction in depressed suicide attempters. Am J Psychiatry 158:735–741, 2001

Keller MB, Hanks DL, Klein DN: Summary of the DSM-IV mood disorders field trial and issue overview. Psychiatr Clin North Am 19:1–28, 1996

Kessler RC, McGonagle KA, Zhao S, et al: Lifetime and 12-month prevalence of DSM-III-R psychiatric disorders in the United States: results from the National Comorbidity Study. Arch Gen Psychiatry 51:8–19, 1994

Lehtinen V, Joukamaa M: Epidemiology of depression: prevalence, risk factors and treatment situation. Acta Psychiatr Scand Suppl 377:7–10, 1994

McDaniel JS, Musselman DL, Proter MR: Depression in patients with cancer. Arch Gen Psychiatry 52:89–99, 1995

Mueller TI, Leon AC: Recovery, chronicity, and levels of psychopathology in major depression. Psychiatr Clin North Am 19:85–102, 1996

Olfson M: Subthreshold psychiatric symptoms in a primary care group practice. Arch Gen Psychiatry 53:880–886, 1996

Petronis KR, Samuels JF, Moscicki EK, et al: An epidemiologic investigation of potential risk factors for suicide attempts. Soc Psychiatry Psychiatr Epidemiol 25:193–199, 1990

Simpson SG, Folstein SE, Meyers DA, et al: Bipolar II: the most common bipolar phenotype? Am J Psychiatry 150:901–903, 1993

Weissman MM, Leaf PJ, Bruce ML: The epidemiology of dysthymia in five communities: rates, risks, comorbidity, and treatment. Am J Psychiatry 145:815–819, 1988

Weissman MM, Bland RC, Canino GJ, et al: Cross-national epidemiology of major depression and bipolar disorder. JAMA 276:293–299, 1996

Young MA, Fogg LF, Schefner WA, et al: Interaction of risk factors in predicting suicide. Am J Psychiatry 151:434–435, 1994

UTSA Libraries (Item Charged)

Patron Group: Undergraduate Student
Due Date: 10/16/2015 04:59 AM
Title: Concise guide to mood disorders
                / Steven L. Dubovsky, Amelia N.
                Dubovsky.
Author: Dubovsky, Steven L.
Call Number: RC537 .D83 2002
Enumeration:
Chronology:
Copy: 1
Barcode: *10000002809299*

Patron Group
Due Date
Title

Author
call Number
cnservation
hronology
pp
arcode

DIAGNOSING MOOD DISORDERS

Attempts to classify depression date back at least to the fourth century B.C., when Hippocrates coined the terms *melancholia* (black bile) and *mania* (to be mad). The independent descriptions in 1854 by two French physicians, Falret and Baillarger, of *folie circulaire* and *la folie à double forme* were the first formal diagnoses of alternating episodes of mania and depression as a single disorder. At the beginning of the twentieth century, Emil Kraepelin differentiated schizophrenia (dementia praecox) from "manic-depressive insanity" (now called bipolar disorder) from "manic-depressive insanity" (now called bipolar disorder) on the basis of a deteriorating course of the former and an episodic course of the latter. Kraepelin (1921) believed that manic-depressive insanity was a single illness that included "periodic and circular insanity," mania, and melancholia, although he also acknowledged that in many cases it was difficult to tell the difference between dementia praecox and manic-depressive insanity. Although many of Kraepelin's observations of the symptoms and course of bipolar mood disorder remain accurate (and are the basis of current diagnostic nomenclature), this condition is now known to reflect a complex group of disorders that share features such as a high rate of recurrence, a greater risk of psychosis, and alternations of mood states but differ in other important respects.

In the United States, in the first edition of DSM (American Psychiatric Association 1952), *psychotic depressive reaction* referred to severe depression that did not have an obvious external precipitant. In DSM-II (American Psychiatric Association 1968), reactive depression (described in the next section of this chapter, "Endogenous and Reactive Depression") was diagnosed as *depressive neurosi* (which would now be called atypical depression). In the absence of a precipitant, a diagnosis of psychotic depressive reaction was made when a single episode occurred, and a diagnosis of manic-depressive psychosis was made when there were recurrent depressive episodes, whether or not the patient met current criteria for psychosis or mania. Alternating depression and elation was called *cyclothymia,* which was classified with the personality disorders on the grounds that it was chronic and was not caused by a specific circumstance. Since the introduction of DSM-III (American Psychiatric Association 1980), mood disorder diagnoses have been based on symptom clusters rather than the presence or absence of an identifiable precipitant, because the presence of a precipitant does not demonstrably affect the course or treatment response of mood disorders.

■ ENDOGENOUS AND REACTIVE DEPRESSION

The classification of depression according to whether a psychosocial precipitant is present is derived from a distinction originally drawn by German descriptive psychiatrists between endogenous (vital or melancholic) and reactive depression. Originally, the term *reactive* referred to depression in which the patient reacted positively to interactions and events, usually implying a milder disorder. As the term was translated into English, however, it came to mean depression that developed in reaction to some external stress, implying an association between internal or external precipitants and milder forms of depression. In DSM-II, this concept was conserved in the term *neurotic depressive reaction.* In later informal diagnostic schemes, milder forms of depression in which mood is more responsive to the environment came to be called *hysteroid dysphoria,* a type of depression with atypical symptoms that occurs in a patient with interpersonal sensitivity and a characterological tendency to dramatize (Shea and Hirschfeld 1996). As used in DSM-III-R (American Psychiatric Association 1987), DSM-IV (American

Psychiatric Association 1994), and DSM-IV-TR (American Psychiatric Association 2000), the term *atypical depression* (atypical depression is a modifier of a major depressive episode) is more or less equivalent to *hysteroid dysphoria* and the modern version of *neurotic depression*.

Atypical depression is distinguished by mood reactivity (i.e., the capacity to be cheered up temporarily by positive interactions or events) as well as by marked anergia (leaden paralysis), sensitivity to rejection, self-pity, a reverse diurnal mood swing (depression is worse later in the day), and reverse vegetative symptoms (e.g., increased instead of decreased appetite and sleep). About 15% of depressive episodes have atypical features. Atypical symptoms are common in bipolar depression, but mood is not as reactive. Atypical depression appears to respond better to monoamine oxidase inhibitors and selective serotonin reuptake inhibitors than to tricyclic antidepressants (see Chapter 4).

The term *endogenous depression* referred in the German literature to depression that was unresponsive to the environment and in the American literature to depression without an identifiable precipitant, of greater severity, with more guilt and loss of interest, and with typical vegetative symptoms such as decreased appetite and sleep, difficulty concentrating, early-morning awakening, and a diurnal mood swing (depression is worse in the morning). In DSM-IV-TR, the melancholic features specifier retains most of the features of endogenous depression, although research suggests that "lack of reactivity" and "distinct quality of depressed mood" consistently predict the full syndrome of melancholic depression (Kendler 1997). Although melancholic or endogenous depression can appear in response to an obvious precipitant, it is more likely to respond to antidepressants than to psychotherapy, and there is a low rate of response to placebo. Melancholic and atypical depression are not necessarily mutually exclusive.

The melancholic subtype of major depression as defined by symptoms rather than precipitant is a more severe form of major depression that is associated with more depressive episodes, more symptoms, more impairment, more help-seeking, and more comorbidity with anxiety disorders and nicotine dependence but that is not qualitatively different from nonmelancholic major depression (Kendler 1997). In twins, the presence of melancholic features in one twin was found to increase the risk of major depression but not necessarily melancholia in the other twin (Kendler 1997), suggesting that melancholia may be a marker of greater genetic loading. Twin studies do not suggest an environmental influence on the probability of melancholia in depressed patients (Kendler 1997).

■ DIAGNOSIS AND DSM-IV-TR

The term *affect* usually refers to the outward and changeable manifestation of a person's emotional tone, whereas *mood* is a more enduring emotional orientation that colors the person's psychology. However, the change from the term *affective disorders* in DSM-III to *mood disorders* in DSM-IV (and DSM-IV-TR) does not imply a reconceptualization of what these disorders primarily involve (i.e., dysregulation of mood or dysregulation of affect); the two terms are used interchangeably in DSM-IV and DSM-IV-TR.

DSM-IV and DSM-IV-TR distinguish between mood episodes and mood disorders. An episode is a period lasting at least 2 weeks, during which enough symptoms occur for full criteria to be met for the disorder. Criteria for a major depressive episode are listed in Table 1–1. Patients with or without a history of mania may have a major depressive episode if they fulfill these criteria, but *major depressive disorder* (MDD) refers to one or more episodes of major depression in the absence of mania or hypomania (i.e., unipolar depression). A major depressive episode may have psychotic, melancholic (Table 1–2), and/or atypical features (Table 1–3).

Familiarity with several common terms facilitates interpretation of studies of mood disorders. *Response* is usually defined as at least 50% improvement, whereas *partial response* is 25%–50% improvement and *nonresponse* is less than 25% improvement. According to this terminology, patients who are half as symptomatic as they were at the beginning of treatment have responded to treatment. This is not a trivial point, given that most studies consider

TABLE 1–1.   **DSM-IV-TR criteria for a major depressive episode**

A. Five (or more) of the following symptoms have been present during the same 2-week period and represent a change from previous functioning; at least one of the symptoms is either (1) depressed mood or (2) loss of interest or pleasure.

Note: Do not include symptoms that are clearly due to a general medical condition, or mood-incongruent delusions or hallucinations.

(1)   depressed mood most of the day, nearly every day, as indicated by either subjective report (e.g., feels sad or empty) or observation made by others (e.g., appears tearful).   **Note:** In children and adolescents, can be irritable mood.

(2)   markedly diminished interest or pleasure in all, or almost all, activities most of the day, nearly every day (as indicated by either subjective account or observation made by others)

(3)   significant weight loss when not dieting or weight gain (e.g., a change of more than 5% of body weight in a month), or decrease or increase in appetite nearly every day.   **Note:** In children, consider failure to make expected weight gains.

(4)   insomnia or hypersomnia nearly every day

(5)   psychomotor agitation or retardation nearly every day (observable by others, not merely subjective feelings of restlessness or being slowed down)

(6)   fatigue or loss of energy nearly every day

(7)   feelings of worthlessness or excessive or inappropriate guilt (which may be delusional) nearly every day (not merely self-reproach or guilt about being sick)

(8)   diminished ability to think or concentrate, or indecisiveness, nearly every day (either by subjective account or as observed by others)

(9)   recurrent thoughts of death (not just fear of dying), recurrent suicidal ideation without a specific plan, or a suicide attempt or a specific plan for committing suicide

B. The symptoms do not meet criteria for a Mixed Episode

C. The symptoms cause clinically significant distress or impairment in social, occupational, or other important areas of functioning.

TABLE 1–1.	**DSM-IV-TR criteria for a major depressive episode** *(continued)*

D. The symptoms are not due to the direct physiological effects of a substance (e.g., a drug of abuse, a medication) or a general medical condition (e.g., hypothyroidism).

E. The symptoms are not better accounted for by Bereavement, i.e., after the loss of a loved one, the symptoms persist for longer than 2 months or are characterized by marked functional impairment, morbid preoccupation with worthlessness, suicidal ideation, psychotic symptoms, or psychomotor retardation.

TABLE 1–2.	**DSM-IV-TR criteria for melancholic features specifier**

Specify if:

With Melancholic Features (can be applied to the current or most recent Major Depressive Episode in Major Depressive Disorder and to a Major Depressive Episode in Bipolar I or Bipolar II Disorder only if it is the most recent type of mood episode)

A. Either of the following, occurring during the most severe period of the current episode:
   (1) loss of pleasure in all, or almost all, activities
   (2) lack of reactivity to usually pleasurable stimuli (does not feel much better, even temporarily, when something good happens)

B. Three (or more) of the following:
   (1) distinct quality of depressed mood (i.e., the depressed mood is experienced as distinctly different from the kind of feeling experienced after the death of a loved one)
   (2) depression regularly worse in the morning
   (3) early morning awakening (at least 2 hours before usual time of awakening)
   (4) marked psychomotor retardation or agitation
   (5) significant anorexia or weight loss
   (6) excessive or inappropriate guilt

TABLE 1–3.　**DSM-IV-TR criteria for atypical features specifier**

Specify if:

   With Atypical Features (can be applied when these features
   predominate during the most recent 2 weeks of a current Major
   Depressive Episode in Major Depressive Disorder or in Bipolar I or
   Bipolar II Disorder when a current Major Depressive Episode is the
   most recent type of mood episode, or when these features predominate
   during the most recent 2 years of Dysthymic Disorder; if the Major
   Depressive Episode is not current, it applies if the feature
   predominates during any 2-week period)

A. Mood reactivity (i.e., mood brightens in response to actual or potential
    positive events)
B. Two (or more) of the following features:
    (1) significant weight gain or increase in appetite
    (2) hypersomnia
    (3) leaden paralysis (i.e., heavy, leaden feelings in arms or legs)
    (4) long-standing pattern of interpersonal rejection sensitivity (not
         limited to episodes of mood disturbance) that results in
         significant social or occupational impairment
C. Criteria are not met for With Melancholic Features or With Catatonic
    Features during the same episode.

---

response rather than remission as the end point. *Remission* is defined as the state of having few or no symptoms of a mood disorder
for at least 8 weeks. *Recovery* has occurred if no symptoms have
been present for more than 8 weeks, implying that the disorder is
quiescent. A *relapse* is a return of symptoms during the period of
remission, which implies continuation of the original episode;
whereas *recurrence* is a later return of symptoms (i.e., during recovery), suggesting that a new episode has developed. These distinctions are easier to make in theory than in clinical practice, where
mild residual symptoms or persistent psychosocial dysfunction are
easily overlooked after improvement of the more dramatic manifestations of an episode, leading to the mistaken conclusion that a return of more severe symptoms represents a new episode rather than

8

an exacerbation of the original episode. It is not yet known whether relapse associated with failure of treatment to produce a complete remission requires a different management strategy than failure to prevent a recurrence of treatment that has been completely effective initially.

■ UNIPOLAR AND BIPOLAR MOOD DISORDERS

One of the most important distinctions between mood disorders is the distinction between unipolar and bipolar categories. Unipolar mood disorders are characterized by depressive symptoms in the absence of a history of a pathologically elevated mood. In bipolar mood disorders, depression alternates or is mixed with mania or hypomania. Patients who have only had recurrent mania ("unipolar mania") are given the diagnosis of bipolar mood disorder, on the assumption that they will eventually have an episode of depression. DSM-IV-TR criteria for a manic episode are listed in Table 1–4. Hypomania is a milder form of pathologically elevated mood that can be present for a shorter period before it is diagnosed; criteria for a hypomanic episode are given in Table 1–5. Although most people think of elation as a defining characteristic of mania and hypomania, many patients experience only irritability, anxiety, or a dysphoric sense of increased energy, as if they were "crawling out of their skins." This kind of presentation may occur most frequently in women and younger patients with bipolar disorder and in antidepressant-induced hypomania. In DSM-IV-TR, mania is described as a state of increased engagement in goal-directed behavior that is pleasurable and has obvious potential for harm. However, manic behavior is frequently disorganized without being consistently directed toward one particular goal, and mental activity may be increased more than physical activity.

It would seem apparent that the bipolar–unipolar distinction is dichotomous: a patient either is or is not manic, and bipolar and unipolar depression often have different features (Table 1–6). On closer scrutiny, these distinctions are not as obvious as they first seem (Dubovsky 1997). For example, unipolar depression can be

TABLE 1–4.	DSM-IV-TR criteria for a manic episode

A. A distinct period of abnormally and persistently elevated, expansive, or irritable mood, lasting at least 1 week (or any duration if hospitalization is necessary).

B. During the period of mood disturbance, three (or more) of the following symptoms have persisted (four if the mood is only irritable) and have been present to a significant degree:

   (1) inflated self-esteem or grandiosity
   (2) decreased need for sleep (e.g., feels rested after only 3 hours of sleep)
   (3) more talkative than usual or pressure to keep talking
   (4) flight of ideas or subjective experience that thoughts are racing
   (5) distractibility (i.e., attention too easily drawn to unimportant or irrelevant external stimuli)
   (6) increase in goal-directed activity (either socially, at work or school, or sexually) or psychomotor agitation
   (7) excessive involvement in pleasurable activities that have a high potential for painful consequences (e.g., engaging in unrestrained buying sprees, sexual indiscretions, or foolish business investments)

C. The symptoms do not meet criteria for a Mixed Episode.

D. The mood disturbance is sufficiently severe to cause marked impairment in occupational functioning or in usual social activities or relationships with others, or to necessitate hospitalization to prevent harm to self or others, or there are psychotic features.

E. The symptoms are not due to the direct physiological effects of a substance (e.g., a drug of abuse, a medication, or other treatment) or a general medical condition (e.g., hyperthyroidism).

Note: Manic-like episodes that are clearly caused by somatic antidepressant treatment (e.g., medication, electroconvulsive therapy, light therapy) should not count toward a diagnosis of Bipolar I Disorder.

psychotic with severe depressive symptoms, and unipolar depressive episodes may be even more recurrent than in bipolar depression, as occurs with recurrent brief depression. Lithium can increase the effectiveness of antidepressants in unipolar depression,

TABLE 1–5. **DSM-IV-TR criteria for a hypomanic episode**

A. A distinct period of persistently elevated, expansive, or irritable mood, lasting throughout at least 4 days, that is clearly different from the usual nondepressed mood.

B. During the period of mood disturbance, three (or more) of the following symptoms have persisted (four if the mood is only irritable) and have been present to a significant degree:

(1) inflated self-esteem or grandiosity

(2) decreased need for sleep (e.g., feels rested after only 3 hours of sleep)

(3) more talkative than usual or pressure to keep talking

(4) flight of ideas or subjective experience that thoughts are racing

(5) distractibility (i.e., attention too easily drawn to unimportant or irrelevant external stimuli)

(6) increase in goal-directed activity (either socially, at work or school, or sexually) or psychomotor agitation

(7) excessive involvement in pleasurable activities that have a high potential for painful consequences (e.g., the person engages in unrestrained buying sprees, sexual indiscretions, or foolish business investments)

C. The episode is associated with an unequivocal change in functioning that is uncharacteristic of the person when not symptomatic.

D. The disturbance in mood and the change in functioning are observable by others.

E. The episode is not severe enough to cause marked impairment in social or occupational functioning, or to necessitate hospitalization, and there are no psychotic features.

F. The symptoms are not due to the direct physiological effects of a substance (e.g., a drug of abuse, a medication, or other treatment) or a general medical condition (e.g., hyperthyroidism).

Note: Hypomanic-like episodes that are clearly caused by somatic antidepressant treatment (e.g., medication, electroconvulsive therapy, light therapy) should not count toward a diagnosis of Bipolar II Disorder.

TABLE 1–6. **Differences between unipolar and bipolar depression**

Unipolar depression	Bipolar depression
Later onset	Earlier onset
Fewer episodes	More episodes
More gradual onset	Acute onset
Female>>male	Female=male
More psychomotor agitation	More psychomotor retardation and lethargy
Typical symptoms	Atypical symptoms
Insomnia	Hypersomnia
Lower risk of suicide	Greater risk of suicide
Less frequently accompanied by psychotic symptoms in younger patients	Greater likelihood of psychotic symptoms in younger patients
Antidepressants more effective	Antidepressants less effective
Lithium less effective	Lithium more effective
Family history of depression	Family history of mania and depression
Normal $[Ca^{2+}]_i$	Increased $[Ca^{2+}]_i$

Note. $[Ca^{2+}]_i$=free intracellular concentration of calcium ions.

and electroconvulsive therapy (ECT) is effective in treating both mania and depression. Patients with unipolar depression may have symptoms generally associated with bipolar disorder such as agitation, racing thoughts, overspending, and grandiose delusions (e.g., the delusion that one is the worst person who ever lived). Unipolar and bipolar disorders can aggregate in the same families, and some studies suggest there are no significant differences between unipolar and bipolar disorder with regard to familial rates of bipolar illness (Winokur 1995); bipolar depression may appear in families with unipolar disorder parents and grandparents. Some of the overlapping features of bipolar and unipolar mood disorders are illustrated in Figure 1–1.

Given that mania and depression are opposite mood states, one would think that only one of the two disorders could be present at a time. However, between 30% and 50% of manic episodes are

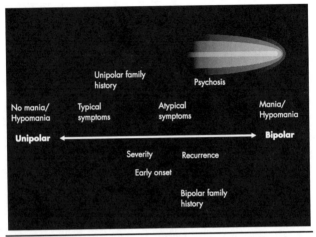

FIGURE 1–1. **Overlap of bipolar and unipolar mood disorders.**

accompanied by depressive symptoms (McElroy et al. 1992). According to DSM-IV-TR, a mixed episode (dysphoric mania) should be diagnosed if the full criteria (except duration) are met for both mania and major depression. However, many more depressed patients have manic symptoms, and manic patients have depressive symptoms, as exemplified by depression accompanied by dramatic behavior, outbursts of rage, and decreased need for sleep, and hypomania accompanied by suicide attempts and fatigue (McElroy et al. 1992). Dysphoric mania is more common among females and is associated with a greater risk of suicide and a poorer response to lithium (McElroy et al. 1992). There may also be an association between mixed states and very rapid mood swings (ultradian cycling).

■ SPECIFIC MOOD DISORDERS

The identification of an episode of mania and/or depression is the first step in making a comprehensive diagnosis. The next steps are

to decide which modifiers in addition to melanchol¹
features apply to the episode and then to consider specific
of mood disorders. Some of these categorical subtypes meet criteria
for DSM-IV-TR mood disorders with or without symptomatic or
course specifiers, and some are commonly recognized syndromes
that may not meet formal diagnostic criteria but are nonetheless
clinically important.

Major Depressive Disorder

MDD is characterized by one or more major depressive episodes in
the absence of mania or hypomania. Depressive syndromes caused
by medical illnesses (mood disorder due to a general medical condition) and by medications or psychoactive substances (substance-
induced mood disorder) are not considered primary mood disorders
and do not qualify for a diagnosis of MDD. In DSM-IV-TR, there
are a number of course specifiers that can be applied to the current
or most recent depressive episode. These course specifiers (severity,
psychosis, degree of remission, chronicity, catatonic features, melancholic features, atypical features, and postpartum onset) are discussed throughout this chapter. DSM-IV-TR provides two additional
descriptors for patients with recurrent depressive episodes: with (or
without) interepisode recovery and with seasonal pattern.

   Although MDD can consist of a single episode, recurrence is
the rule rather than the exception. After a single major depressive
episode, the risk of a second episode is around 50%; after a third episode, the risk of a fourth is around 90% (Thase 1990). Each new
episode tends to occur sooner and more abruptly, and new episodes
often include the same symptoms that previous episodes included,
along with new and more severe symptoms. The tendency to accelerate and become more complex is characteristic of all mood disorders.

   DSM-IV-TR specifiers indicate whether a major depressive episode has remitted fully (i.e., no symptoms for at least 2 months),
partially (i.e., not enough ongoing depressive symptoms to qualify
for a diagnosis of a major depressive episode, or no symptoms for

less than 2 months), or not at all (i.e., a chronic major depressive episode). Longitudinal course specifiers for MDD indicate whether recurrent major depressive episodes remit completely or partially in between episodes and whether major depressive episodes are superimposed on dysthymia. The degree of remission and of premorbid depression can be difficult to determine when less severe residual symptoms are overlooked, because the patient no longer feels severely depressed. It can also be difficult to decide whether certain traits or ways of thinking are residual depressive symptoms. For example, globally negative thinking, all-or-nothing assumptions such as "If everyone doesn't accept me all the time, no one cares about me at all" or "If I make a mistake, I'm totally incompetent," and chronic joylessness, crankiness, or interpersonal hypersensitivity may be symptoms of subsyndromal residual depression that require more aggressive treatment and that left untreated may predispose to relapse or recurrence of the full syndrome.

Masked Depression

As many as 50% of major depressive episodes are unrecognized because a depressed mood is less obvious than other symptoms of the disorder. Alexithymia, or the inability to express emotions in words, can lead to manifestation of depressed mood as physical symptoms of depression—such as insomnia, low energy, and difficulty concentrating—without any awareness of feeling depressed. Minor physical dysfunction may be magnified by hypervigilance for anything that feels dangerous or bad, making it difficult to distinguish chronic major depression from somatization disorder and hypochondriasis. Substance use as a form of self-treatment for depression can be more obvious than the underlying mood disorder. When pathological character traits are intensified in response to an underlying mood disorder, a personality disorder may seem to be the primary problem. Additional common masked presentations of major depression include marital and family conflicts, absenteeism from work, poor school performance, social withdrawal, loss of a sense of humor, and lack of motivation.

Many depressed patients have mild cognitive dysfunction that improves with encouragement. However, some depressed patients have a pattern of subcortical dementia that may be indistinguishable from primary dementia. In older patients and patients with preexisting mild dementia, depression may be expressed mainly as cognitive dysfunction, the disturbance in mood being masked by aprosodia (described later in this section). The term *depressive pseudodementia* is often used to describe this presentation, but a more accurate term would be *dementia syndrome of depression* or *reversible dementia of depression.* There may be a neurological component to depressive dementia, as is suggested by an association of global brain atrophy and white matter lesions with greater levels of cognitive impairment in depressed patients who do not have obvious neurological disease (Soares and Mann 1997).

The dementia syndrome of depression may be found on close questioning to be accompanied by changes in energy, appetite, and sleep and a family history of depression, but not necessarily obvious changes in mood. The only way to be confident that depression is not the cause of apparent dementia may be to observe the patient's response to an antidepressant. However, a majority of patients whose depressive dementias remit partially or completely with antidepressant treatment are found on follow-up to develop primary dementia that no longer responds to antidepressants (Reynolds and Hoch 1987). One explanation for this outcome is that the effect of depression on subcortical structures lowers the threshold for the expression of coexisting early dementia that would otherwise not be recognizable for some time. With successful treatment of the depression, dementia is no longer apparent, but as dementia progresses, it becomes severe enough to be identifiable in its own right. In other cases, depression may be a prodromal symptom of dementia. Even in these cases, treatment of depression can delay the onset of obvious irreversible primary dementia.

Another form of masked depression encountered in neurological settings occurs in patients with aprosodia. Aprosodia, or loss of the capacity to convey or understand emotional and other nuances of speech and behavior (prosody), is a manifestation of disease of the nondominant hemisphere. Patients with aprosodia lose the capacity to understand, repeat, or communicate emotional meaning, even when speech remains intact. If they become depressed, such patients may not appear or feel sad or unhappy, but their thoughts and actions are derivatives of a depressive orientation. For example, affect may be irritable or blunted rather than depressed. Negativistic behavior (e.g., mutism, gross noncompliance with medical therapy, refusal to eat), withdrawal, catatonia, or violent outbursts may be much more obvious than depressed mood. Vegetative symptoms such as disturbances of appetite, energy, and sleep may appear to be symptoms of the neurological illness. However, treatment with an antidepressant or ECT can produce dramatic improvement.

Chronic Depression

Chronic forms of depression account for 12%–35% of depressive disorders (Scott 1988). Rates of chronicity in depression vary with the comprehensiveness of the evaluation that is performed (Scott 1988). More patients meet criteria for chronicity when it is defined by the presence of any depressive symptoms than when it is defined as a level of symptomatology that is above some definite level, such as a Hamilton Rating Scale for Depression (Ham-D) score of 10. Even after remission of specific depressive symptoms, many patients continue to experience family dysfunction, occupational impairment, and poor physical health (Thase 1992). If chronic depression is defined in part by impaired functioning, some of these patients may be considered chronically depressed even if specific depressive symptoms are not obvious.

Dysthymic Disorder

Dysthymic disorder (*dysthymia* means "ill-tempered") was introduced in DSM-III to indicate chronic depression that was less severe than major depression. The cardinal feature of dysthymic disorder is a chronically depressed mood that is present most of the day, more days than not, for at least 2 years. The concept of dysthymic disorder as mild, chronic depression began with diagnoses in earlier versions of DSM such as chronic depression and depressive personality, and this concept has continued to evolve. For example, in the change from DSM-III to DSM-III-R, 8 symptoms were deleted, an appetite disturbance was added, and descriptions of some symptoms were reworded so that the number of associated symptoms was decreased from 13 to 6. In addition, the minimum number of symptoms required for a diagnosis of dysthymic disorder was reduced from 3 to 2. These changes did not affect the number of adults who meet criteria for dysthymic disorder (Gwirtsman et al. 1997); it is not known whether the number of patients with adolescent- or geriatric-onset dysthymia remains unchanged (Gwirtsman et al. 1997).

DSM-IV-TR criteria for dysthymic disorder (Table 1–7) are essentially the same as DSM-III-R criteria, the primary changes being the addition of an impairment criterion and the elimination of a distinction between primary and secondary dysthymia. In an attempt to distinguish between chronic MDD and dysthymic disorder, DSM-IV-TR stipulates that chronic depressive symptoms lasting less than 2 years after a major depressive episode and otherwise meeting criteria for dysthymic disorder be diagnosed as a major depressive episode in partial remission; if a full remission from a major depressive episode lasts at least 6 months and is then followed by dysthymia, a diagnosis of dysthymic disorder is justified.

What is the real difference between MDD and dysthymic disorder? Dysthymia begins insidiously and must be present for at least 2 years, during which time criteria cannot be met for a major depressive episode (First et al. 1996). However, retrospective accounts of the onset of a mood disorder years in the past are likely to be colored by patients' moods at the time of recall, making anything but prospective independent evaluation of patients who are at risk for depression unreliable in distinguishing between dysthymic disorder and chronic MDD.

Another defining difference is that more depressive symptoms are required for a diagnosis of MDD than for a diagnosis of dysthymic disorder. However, as Table 1–8 shows, if a dysthymic patient reports only two more symptoms, the diagnosis is changed to MDD.

TABLE 1–7. **DSM-IV-TR criteria for dysthymic disorder**

A. Depressed mood for most of the day, for more days than not, as indicated either by subjective account or observation by others, for at least 2 years. **Note:** In children and adolescents, mood can be irritable and duration must be at least 1 year.

B. Presence, while depressed, of two (or more) of the following:
   (1) poor appetite or overeating
   (2) insomnia or hypersomnia
   (3) low energy or fatigue
   (4) low self-esteem
   (5) poor concentration or difficulty making decisions
   (6) feelings of hopelessness

C. During the 2-year period (1 year for children or adolescents) of the disturbance, the person has never been without the symptoms in Criteria A and B for more than 2 months at a time.

D. No Major Depressive Episode has been present during the first 2 years of the disturbance (1 year for children and adolescents); i.e., the disturbance is not better accounted for by chronic Major Depressive Disorder, or Major Depressive Disorder, In Partial Remission.

   Note: There may have been a previous Major Depressive Episode provided there was a full remission (no significant signs or symptoms for 2 months) before development of the Dysthymic Disorder. In addition, after the initial 2 years (1 year in children or adolescents) of Dysthymic Disorder, there may be superimposed episodes of Major Depressive Disorder, in which case both diagnoses may be given when the criteria are met for a Major Depressive Episode.

E. There has never been a Manic Episode, a Mixed Episode, or a Hypomanic Episode, and criteria have never been met for Cyclothymic Disorder.

F. The disturbance does not occur exclusively during the course of a chronic Psychotic Disorder, such as Schizophrenia or Delusional Disorder.

G. The symptoms are not due to the direct physiological effects of a substance (e.g., a drug of abuse, a medication) or a general medical condition (e.g., hypothyroidism).

TABLE 1–7. **DSM-IV-TR criteria for dysthymic disorder** *(continued)*

H. The symptoms cause clinically significant distress or impairment in social, occupational, or other important areas of functioning.

Specify if:

Early Onset: if onset is before age 21 years
Late Onset: if onset is age 21 years or older

Specify (for most recent 2 years of Dysthymic Disorder):

With Atypical Features

This is a common outcome because most patients who meet criteria for dysthymic disorder exhibit more than the minimum number of symptoms required for the diagnosis, regardless of the diagnostic criteria used (e.g., DSM-III, DSM-III-R, or DSM-IV criteria or DSM-IV alternative criteria). Indeed, 80% of patients with dysthymia also have a lifetime diagnosis of major depression, and most patients with dysthymic disorder seek treatment for superimposed major depression (Keller et al. 1996). If a patient has barely the requisite number of symptoms to meet criteria for MDD, does a different disorder exist if the number of symptoms is less a few days later as the disorder inevitably fluctuates? Does the advent of one more symptom in a dysthymic patient mean that the patient now has another illness requiring a different treatment? Is there any difference between severe dysthymia and mild major depression?

TABLE 1–8. **Dysthymic disorder and major depressive disorder compared**

Dysthymic disorder	Major depressive disorder
2 years	2 weeks
Depressed mood	Depressed mood
2 additional symptoms	4 additional symptoms
More cognitive symptoms	More vegetative symptoms
Mild onset may be followed after 2 years by major depression	Onset may be accompanied by more severe symptoms

Compared with dysthymic disorder, MDD does appear to be associated with greater loss of interest or pleasure; loss of appetite and weight; trouble thinking, concentrating, or making decisions; reductions in activity levels; feelings of worthlessness; diurnal mood swing; fatigue or loss of energy; hopelessness; and social withdrawal, which suggests that major depression is a more severe condition, at least with regard to current symptoms (Keller et al. 1996). Conversely, cognitive and social-motivational symptoms have been reported to be more frequent in dysthymic disorder (Klein et al. 1996). Patients with MDD obviously have more depressive symptoms than do patients with dysthymic disorder, because more symptoms are required for a diagnosis of MDD to be made, but there are no substantive qualitative differences in symptomatology between the two conditions (Klein et al. 1996). Patients with MDD usually have higher scores on the Ham-D than do patients with dysthymic disorder, but the difference is not great (Kocsis 1993).

When severity is examined from the standpoint of functioning rather than number of symptoms, the distinction between MDD and dysthymic disorder becomes even less reliable. Dysthymic disorder produces as much impairment as MDD in work, leisure activities, relationships, general health, and ability to perform social roles (Frances 1993). Even minor depression (a Research Diagnostic Criteria [RDC] condition in which the number of depressive symptoms is insufficient to meet criteria for dysthymic disorder or MDD) is associated with almost as much impairment as dysthymic disorder and MDD. Comorbidity with other Axis I disorders and with personality disorders is equally frequent in the two conditions (Kocsis 1993). Despite dysthymic disorder's being defined as a less severe condition, the prognosis of the disorder is not substantially different from that of MDD. Most important, both disorders respond to the same antidepressant and psychotherapeutic regimens (Frances 1993; Scott 1992).

Chronic MDD and dysthymic disorder may be related to each other in a variety of ways. One possibility is that they are separate disorders with overlapping symptoms and with a high rate of comorbidity with each other, with a number of other conditions (such as anxiety, substance-related, eating, somatoform, and personality disorders), and with chronic medical illnesses. Another possibility is that dysthymic disorder is a prodromal phase of MDD, a theory that is suggested by the observation that childhood-onset dysthymic disorder does not persist into adulthood in its original form but is replaced by recurrent MDD and bipolar disorder (Frances 1993). Or both disorders may be different presentations over time of the same disturbance of mood, personality traits, and psychosocial functioning, combining chronic low-grade or residual depression with intermittent recurrence of more severe depression.

In the DSM-IV field trials, patients who met criteria for dysthymia also reported, on average, two-thirds of the symptoms listed in Table 1–9 (Keller et al. 1996). Some of these symptoms are attenuated versions of typical depressive symptoms, whereas others describe global ways of thinking about oneself that overlap with personality traits. A consensus panel for DSM-IV-TR concluded that dysphoria or gloominess for at least 2 years (in adults) or 1 year (in children), along with at least three of six depressive symptoms that include depressive attitudes and behaviors (Gwirtsman et al. 1997) (as opposed to two of four symptoms in DSM-IV), is required for a diagnosis of dysthymic disorder (Table 1–10). Uncertainty about the ways in which dysthymic disorder is distinguished from MDD probably reflects the fluctuating nature of all forms of chronic depression and the frequency with which chronic depression is integrated with personality traits.

TABLE 1–9. **Symptoms endorsed by patients meeting DSM-IV criteria for dysthymic disorder**

Low self-esteem, feelings of inadequacy
Pessimism, despair, or hopelessness
Social withdrawal
Chronic fatigue or tiredness
Guilt, brooding about the past
Irritability, excessive anger
Decreased activity, effectiveness, or productivity
Difficulty thinking: poor concentration, poor memory, indecisiveness
Generalized loss of interest or pleasure (mild anhedonia)

TABLE 1–10. **DSM-IV-TR alternative research criteria B for dysthymic disorder**

B.   Presence, while depressed, of three (or more) of the following:

 (1) low self-esteem or self-confidence, or feelings of inadequacy
 (2) feelings of pessimism, despair, or hopelessness
 (3) generalized loss of interest or pleasure
 (4) social withdrawal
 (5) chronic fatigue or tiredness
 (6) feelings of guilt, brooding about the past
 (7) subjective feelings of irritability or excessive anger
 (8) decreased activity, effectiveness, or productivity
 (9) difficulty in thinking, reflected by poor concentration, poor memory, or indecisiveness

---

Minor Depression

Minor depressive disorder is an RDC diagnosis in which the most prominent disturbance is a sustained depressed mood, without the full depressive syndrome (Keller et al. 1996). The RDC for minor depression include feeling depressed or down in the dumps for 1 week (probable minor depression) or 2 weeks (definite minor depression) (Keller et al. 1996). For a diagnosis to be made, the patient must have at least two symptoms on a larger symptom list than the list of DSM-IV-TR criteria for MDD; this larger list includes pessimistic attitude and self-pity and does not include impairment or help-seeking. Minor depression may be chronic, and, like dysthymic disorder, it may be complicated by superimposed major depressive episodes (Keller et al. 1996). Despite its similarity to dysthymia, minor depression is not frequently diagnosed in the United States (Keller et al. 1996).

Double Depression

Although it is not a separate DSM-IV-TR diagnosis, double depression, or dysthymic disorder with a superimposed major depressive episode, has been extensively discussed in the literature, and clinicians use the term frequently. The major depressive episode must appear 2 years or more (1 year in children and adolescents) after the onset of dysthymia for double depression to be formally diagnosed. Double depression is far from uncommon among dysthymic patients. Between 68% and 90% of dysthymic patients experience at least one major depressive episode (Thase 1992), and 25%–50% of patients with MDD have coexisting dysthymic disorder (Hirschfeld 1994). It has been estimated that 22%–66% of all patients with unipolar depression have experienced a combination of dysthymia and major depression (Hirschfeld 1994). A 9-year prospective study found dysthymic disorder with superimposed MDD or recurrent brief depression in 3% of the general population (Hirschfeld 1994).

Compared with episodic MDD (major depressive episodes alternating with euthymia), MDD superimposed on dysthymia has an earlier onset of major depression, is more treatment resistant, and is associated with more severe depressive symptoms, more psychosocial impairment, a greater risk of suicide, and more comorbidity, especially with avoidant and dependent personality disorders (Angst and Wicki 1991; Belsher and Costello 1988). The major depressive episode in double depression is less likely to remit than the major depressive episode in episodic MDD (i.e., recurrent major depression not superimposed on dysthymia) and is more likely to recur. In one study, the relapse rate of major depression after 8 weeks of recovery was 30% for double depression and 4% for episodic MDD (Belsher and Costello 1988). In that study, major depression recurred after 1 year in 50% of patients with double depression and 35% of patients with episodic MDD, and after 2 years in 65% and 37%, respectively. The risk of a bipolar outcome also appears greater in double depression: 29% of patients with double depression in the NIMH-CS developed hypomania, compared with 9% of patients with episodic MDD (Keller 1994).

Subsyndromal Depression

Subsyndromal disorders are conditions that do not meet full diagnostic criteria for particular disorders. Some subsyndromal forms of unipolar depression, such as the RDC condition minor depressive disorder, have formal diagnostic criteria, and even though impairment or seeking treatment is not required for the diagnosis, they are associated with clinically important functional impairment (Keller et al. 1996). In the Epidemiologic Catchment Area study, one-third of people using mental health services had subsyndromal mood disorders (Gwirtsman et al. 1997). There is less certainty about the degree to which some constellations of personality traits may also represent subsyndromal forms of chronic depression.

The concept of a depressive temperament representing either a subsyndromal form of depression expressed through the personality or a "fundamental state" from which more severe depressive episodes emerge later in life was proposed early in the twentieth century by Emil Kraepelin and again in the middle of the century by Kurt Schneider. These and other investigators noted that depression is predictably associated with such personality traits as persistent gloominess or despondency, seriousness, guilt, lack of self-confidence, self-denial, conscientiousness, introversion, and neuroticism (Shea and Hirschfeld 1996). The question that remains to be formally answered is whether such traits are partial expressions of a depressive disorder, manifestations of mildly pathological personality traits mobilized in response to an underlying mood disorder that is then overshadowed by the overexpressed personality traits, or markers of a propensity to develop full syndromal mood disorders later in life.

Akiskal (1991) divided syndromes marked by depressive traits into *subaffective dysthymia,* in which depressive personality traits are caused by chronic subclinical depression, and *character spectrum disorder,* which he considered a type of personality disorder in which depressed mood is just one feature of a chronically unhappy and unfulfilled orientation of the personality. As a result of deliberations by the DSM-IV Personality Disorders Work Group, a version of character spectrum disorder is included in the appendix to DSM-IV-TR as *depressive personality disorder.* The DSM-IV field trials suggested that this condition (Table 1–11) is associated with a passive, unassertive style, in the absence of current diagnosable dys-

TABLE 1–11.	**DSM-IV-TR research criteria for depressive personality disorder**

A.   A pervasive pattern of depressive cognitions and behaviors beginning by early adulthood and present in a variety of contexts, as indicated by five (or more) of the following:
   (1) usual mood is dominated by dejection, gloominess, cheerlessness, joylessness, unhappiness
   (2) self-concept centers around beliefs of inadequacy, worthlessness, and low self-esteem
   (3) is critical, blaming, and derogatory toward self
   (4) is brooding and given to worry
   (5) is negativistic, critical, and judgmental toward others
   (6) is pessimistic
   (7) is prone to feeling guilty or remorseful

B.   Does not occur exclusively during Major Depressive Episodes and is not better accounted for by Dysthymic Disorder.

thymia, in almost 50% of cases. Patients thought to have depressive personality disorder were noted to have a tendency to develop dysthymic disorder or MDD after the diagnosis of depressive personality disorder was made, which suggests that the apparent personality disorder might be an early-onset, traitlike variant or prodrome of a depressive disorder. This hypothesis is supported by the existence of a familial association between depressive personality disorder and other depressive disorders and by the fact that onset is earlier and more depressive episodes occur in patients with MDD and premorbid depressive personalities than in patients with major depression and without these premorbid temperaments (Cassano et al. 1992).

From a clinical standpoint, defining a personality disorder that overlaps with but is distinct from primary mood disorders has the theoretical benefit of identifying a group of patients who would be expected to have poor responses to typical treatments for depression and better responses to specialized psychotherapeutic approaches. However, the overlap between abnormal mood and stable personality traits is often so extensive that the two can be indistinguishable

(Shea and Hirschfeld 1996). As a result, many people with diagnoses of MDD and/or dysthymia meet DSM-IV symptomatic criteria for depressive personality disorder. In one study, 41% of patients with a major depressive episode were found to meet all criteria for depressive personality disorder, including persistence of symptoms when the full mood disorder was not present (Shea and Hirschfeld 1996).

The impact of an abnormal mood on thinking and behavior can be so profound that it distorts most assessments of personality, making it impossible to determine the degree to which a personality disorder is present in patients with an active primary mood disorder. Chronically unstable or depressed mood can intensify pathological defenses and can skew the ways in which a person experiences the self and others. On personality inventories, depressed people resemble each other more than they resemble themselves when they are not depressed (Hirschfeld et al. 1989). In several studies, more than 50% of patients (or their relatives) with a diagnosis of borderline personality disorder were found to develop major depression, mania, or hypomania or to commit suicide (Akiskal 1991). This finding could indicate a high rate of comorbidity, or it could mean that a substantial number of patients with personality disorder diagnoses actually have state-dependent exacerbation of pathological personality traits by a covert mood disorder. Because mild depressive symptoms as well as social impairment can persist after remission of a full depressive syndrome, persistent passivity, negative thinking, low self-esteem, cynicism, and related traits in the absence of a diagnosable mood disorder could represent residual symptoms of a previous episode or prodromal symptoms of another episode, rather than a true personality disorder. In the absence of any validated method for distinguishing the two, the most prudent approach for the clinician is to treat depression as vigorously as possible before diagnosing a personality disorder. However, even though features such as negative therapeutic reactions, attachment to a negative view of the self and others, self-destructive motivations, and treatment nonadherence are not necessarily diagnostic of a personality disorder, such tendencies often must be addressed because they frequently interfere with a positive response to even the most straightforward antidepressant regimen.

Psychotic Depression

The term *psychotic depression* (or *delusional depression*) refers to a major depressive episode accompanied by psychotic features (i.e., delusions and/or hallucinations). Some clinicians believe that psychotic depression is relatively uncommon. However, most studies continue to demonstrate that 16%–54% of depressed patients have psychotic symptoms, the incidence of psychosis being higher in depressed inpatients (Dubovsky and Thomas 1992). Delusions occur without hallucinations in one-half to two-thirds of adults with psychotic depression, whereas hallucinations are unaccompanied by delusions in 3%–25% of patients (Dubovsky and Thomas 1992). Half of all psychotically depressed patients experience more than one kind of delusion (Dubovsky and Thomas 1992). Hallucinations occur more frequently than delusions in younger depressed patients and in patients with bipolar psychotic depression. The common belief that visual and olfactory hallucinations are signs of neurological disease has been contradicted by clinical experience with psychotic depression, which demonstrates that auditory and visual hallucinations are equally frequent in psychotic depression and that olfactory and haptic hallucinations may occur in the absence of central nervous system disease, especially in patients with bipolar depression (Dubovsky and Thomas 1992).

The classification of psychotic symptoms as mood congruent (i.e., consistent with a depressed or elated mood) or mood incongruent is complex. Prominent mood-incongruent psychotic symptoms in depressed patients such as delusions of control, along with poor adolescent adjustment, may be associated with a somewhat worse prognosis of psychotic depression (Tsuang and Coryell 1993). The RDC, which were used in many earlier studies of psychotic depression, specify a diagnosis of schizoaffective disorder for depressed patients with mood-incongruent psychotic features. However, psychotic bipolar depression is frequently associated with mood-incongruent psychotic symptoms, some of which may be bizarre and easily mistaken for typical "schizophrenic" symptoms; a formal thought disorder occurs in at least 20% of bipolar psychotically depressed patients (Goodwin and Jamison 1991). Because bipolar illness is overrepresented in psychotic depression, it may be bipolar illness and not mood incongruence that contributes to a poorer treatment response in mood-incongruent psychotic depression. In recognition of the uncertain contribution of mood incongruence to prognosis, DSM-IV-TR requires the existence of psychotic symptoms for 2 or more weeks in the absence of prominent mood symptoms for a diagnosis of schizoaffective disorder, a specifier that, along with poor adolescent adjustment, seems more consistently associated with a poorer prognosis of mixed affective and psychotic syndromes than the RDC (Coryell 1996), although persistent subsyndromal affective symptoms (e.g., changes in sleep or energy) may be overlooked when psychotic symptoms are more obvious.

Recognizing psychotic symptoms in depressed patients is not always straightforward. If the patient does not seem severely depressed (this can occur in patients with psychotic bipolar depression in whom elevated mood and energy mixed with depression make them appear less depressed than they feel), the clinician might not inquire about psychotic symptoms. Some patients do not consider hearing voices, seeing things, paranoia, or ideas of reference to be abnormal and do not report such symptoms. Other patients conceal psychotic symptoms because they do not want to be considered "crazy." To be certain that psychotic symptoms are not present, it may be necessary to ask repeatedly about them, beginning with nonspecific questions such as "Does your mind ever play tricks on you?" and progressing gradually to more specific questions such as "Do you ever hear your name called when there's no one there?" and then "Do you ever hear a voice saying more than your name?" Rather than asking first about ideas of persecution, the clinician might ask, "Do you ever feel so self-conscious that it seems that people are staring at you?" and then "Do you ever get the feeling of being watched or followed?"

Psychotic features often emerge after several episodes of non-psychotic depression. Once psychotic symptoms occur, they reappear with each subsequent episode, even if depression in later episodes is not as severe. With each recurrence, psychotic symptoms take the same form that they did in previous episodes (e.g., patients with hallucinations have them in the same modality and with the same content from episode to episode) (Dubovsky and Thomas 1992). Relatives of psychotically depressed patients have an increased risk of psychotic depression as well as other psychotic disorders such as schizophrenia, and when psychotic depression is present, the content of the psychosis tends to be similar to that of the psychosis experienced by the proband.

Whereas treatment with both an antipsychotic drug and an antidepressant is usually necessary for remission of psychotic depression, antipsychotic drugs may improve the depression and the antidepressant may improve the psychosis (Dubovsky and Thomas 1992). This fact, and the additional observation of aggregation of both mood disorders and schizophrenia in families of patients with psychotic depression, suggests that psychotic depression is not a simple combination of psychosis and depression but rather a complex interaction between the capacity to become psychotic and the capacity to become depressed (Dubovsky and Thomas 1992). Depression may have to reach a certain level of severity for psychosis to be expressed for the first time, but once psychosis develops, a unique disorder has evolved. Features in addition to the unique treatment response that distinguish psychotic from nonpsychotic depression include a greater rate of recurrence; a higher suicide risk; a higher rate of nonsuppression on the dexamethasone suppression test, with higher cortisol levels after administration of dexamethasone; more prominent sleep abnormalities; a level of neuropsychological impairment similar to that seen in schizophrenia; and higher ventricle-to-brain ratios (Coryell 1996; Dubovsky and Thomas 1992). Studies have not yet addressed the extent to which the symptomatology, course, and treatment response of psychotic depression are a function of psychosis itself or the overrepresentation of bipolar disorder in psychotically depressed patients.

Involutional Depression

Estimates of the prevalence of major depression among elderly people range from 2%–4% in community samples to 12% among medically hospitalized older patients to 16% among geriatric patients in long-term care (Blazer and Koenig 1996). Late-onset depression is associated with an increased likelihood of cerebrovascular disease and enlarged ventricles and, in younger patients, may be more likely than depression to be accompanied by prominent cognitive complaints. First onset of unipolar depression in elderly patients is often associated with cerebrovascular disease, especially on the left side of the brain (whereas late-onset mania is often associated with right-sided disease). Contrary to popular wisdom, depression in women does not begin at the time of menopause, although depression tends to recur over the years with each reproductive event (e.g., menarche, childbirth, menopause) (Dell and Stewart 2000). Because of the likelihood of associated neurological impairment, depression that appears for the first time in a geriatric patient is more difficult to treat than depression that begins earlier in life.

Postpartum Depression

In contrast to postpartum "blues," which occur in as many as 85% of new mothers and last no longer than 2 weeks, postpartum depression occurs in about 10% of mothers and is much less likely to remit without treatment. Risk factors for postpartum depression include a patient or family history of a mood disorder, unwanted pregnancy, maternal unemployment, a dysfunctional relationship with the child's father, inadequate social support, lack of breast-feeding, and the mother as head of the household; in addition, postpartum depression increases the chance of alcohol and illicit drug use among teenage mothers. Depressed mothers of preschoolers have more negative perceptions of and more negative interactions with their children, and there is some evidence that depression in a mother adversely affects temperament and cognitive development in her infant (Beck 1996). Depression that begins for the first time in the postpartum period is more likely to have a bipolar outcome; postpartum psychosis very frequently is a manifestation of bipolar disorder. There is a 50% chance of recurrence of postpartum psychosis in bipolar disorder patients (Rohde and Manerous 1992).

Recurrent Brief Depression

The RDC and the DSM-IV-TR criteria are in agreement that 2 weeks of continuous symptoms are required for a diagnosis of a major depressive episode to be made. Jules Angst described a depressive disorder called *recurrent brief depression* in which depressive episodes meet DSM-IV symptomatic but not duration criteria for major depression (Angst and Hochstrasser 1994). Depressive episodes in recurrent brief depression have the same number and severity of symptoms as DSM-IV major depressive episodes but last 1 day to 1 week. Depressive episodes must recur at least once per month over at least 12 months (not in association with the menstrual cycle) for recurrent brief depression to be diagnosed (Angst and Hochstrasser 1994). Although each acute depressive episode is short-lived, recurrent brief depression carries a high risk of suicide (Lepine et al. 1995), perhaps because of the inevitable return of depression and the repeated drastic contrast between the depressed and well states.

In the DSM-IV mood disorders field trial, 1.5% of 524 subjects had a lifetime history of recurrent brief depression, and the 1-year prevalence of recurrent brief depressive disorder was 7% (Keller et al. 1996). Recurrent brief depression and MDD have been found to have similar rates of comorbidity with panic disorder, generalized anxiety disorder, and substance use disorders (Keller et al. 1996). Recurrent brief depression has also been found often to have a seasonal pattern, with more recurrences in the winter (Keller et al. 1996).

One might assume that such a highly recurrent mood disorder would be apt eventually to have a bipolar outcome, and in fact, prophylaxis of brief depressive recurrences is more successful with lithium than with antidepressants (Angst et al. 1990). However, extended follow-up of patients with this condition demonstrates that they never develop mania or hypomania (Angst and Hochstrasser 1994; Angst et al. 1990). This important observation suggests that recurrence may be a feature of mood disorders that is more common in, but not restricted to, bipolar subtypes and that lithium therapy may be an antirecurrence as much as an antimanic treatment. The latter point is supported by the capacity of lithium to prevent recurrences of other cyclical and recurrent disorders such as cluster headaches.

■ BIPOLAR SUBTYPES

Bipolar disorder is defined by episodes of mania and/or hypomania (DSM-IV-TR criteria for manic and hypomanic episodes are given in Tables 1–4 and 1–5). DSM-IV-TR includes two primary subtypes of bipolar disorder. Bipolar I disorder is characterized by manic episodes with or without episodes of hypomania. In bipolar II disorder, one or more hypomanic episodes occur but the patient never experiences mania. Hypomanic episodes tend to be milder than bipolar II depressive episodes. Evidence that bipolar II disorder is distinct from bipolar I disorder comes from several sources (Akiskal 1996). Patients with bipolar II disorder never become manic, despite multiple hypomanic episodes. In addition, the bipolar II diagnosis seems to "breed true," in that patients with this diagnosis have relatives with hypomania but not mania, whereas patients with bipolar I disorder have some relatives who have had mania and some who have had only hypomania. Rapid cycling, which is described later (see "Rapid Cycling"), seems to be more common in bipolar II disorder.

Although bipolar III disorder is not a DSM-IV-TR diagnosis, the term has been used in connection with patients with a history of depression who have at least one blood relative with a history of mania, on the grounds that such patients may have a bipolar diathesis that has not yet been expressed. In some circles, *bipolar III* refers to antidepressant-induced mania and *bipolar IV* is used to describe the condition of depressed patients with a family history of mania. In DSM-IV-TR, mania or hypomania that appears in response to treatment with an antidepressant is not counted toward a diagnosis of a primary bipolar mood disorder, but many clinicians consider antidepressant-induced mania to be an indication of the capacity to develop mania or hypomania spontaneously and there-fore a sign of a type of bipolar mood disorder (this seems most likely to be true of children and adolescents) (Akiskal 1995).

Brief Hypomania

Angst (1995) defined a subtype of hypomania called *brief hypomania.* Brief hypomania is characterized by the same symptoms as hy-pomania, but the duration of symptoms is 1–3 days, rather than the 4 or more days required by DSM-IV-TR for a diagnosis of hypoma-nia. Angst found that despite the short duration of any episode, brief hypomania has a very high rate of recurrence and produces marked impairment. In one study, the prevalence of brief hypomania was 2.28% among patients with bipolar mood disorders (Angst 1995), but further data are needed before it can be stated that brief hypo-mania is a distinct disorder and not a manifestation of bipolar II dis-order. Ultrarapid (ultradian) cycling, which is discussed in "Rapid Cycling," probably would qualify as a condition associated with manic or hypomanic symptoms lasting hours to a day or two but recurring very frequently. It is not known whether brief hypomania is characterized by euthymia between hypomanic episodes.

Bipolar Depression

Depression in patients with bipolar mood disorders may alternate or be mixed with mania. Bipolar depression that is not mixed with hy-pomania is characterized by "atypical" symptoms such as hyper-somnia, anergia, carbohydrate craving, and psychomotor slowing. However, in contrast to atypical unipolar depression, mood in bipo-lar depression that is not mixed with hypomania is usually not reac-tive. Especially in younger patients, bipolar depression is associated with psychotic symptoms more frequently than is unipo-lar depression (Mitchell et al. 2001). Much of the time, depression and mania are not neatly differentiated states. Depressive symptoms are often mixed with dysphoric hypomanic symptoms such as anxiety, racing thoughts, insomnia, and exquisite interpersonal sensitivity.

Cyclothymic Disorder

Cyclothymic disorder (cyclothymia) was originally classified as a personality disorder with mood swings that are not clearly manic or depressed. Although most investigators now consider cyclothymic disorder a mood disorder, it is still called cyclothymic personality in the RDC. As Table 1–12 indicates, patients with recurrent hypomanic and depressive symptoms that do not reach the threshold for diagnosis of major depression or hypomania may meet DSM-IV-TR criteria for cyclothymia. In the RDC, cyclothymia is characterized by recurrent depressed mood lasting several days, alternating with elevated mood with at least two hypomanic symptoms. In both schemes, the patient rarely experiences a normal mood.

Patients with cyclothymia typically experience unstable mood states lasting days, weeks, or months that alternate between depression, irritability, cheerfulness, and relative normality (Jamison 1996). Many complain of unpredictable changes in energy, vague physical symptoms, and a seasonal pattern of mood swings (e.g., depression in the winter). In some studies, 44% of cyclothymic patients develop hypomania while taking antidepressants, and about one-third experience full-blown hypomanic, manic, or depressive episodes during drug-free follow-up. In addition, at least one-third of the time, the onset of clear bipolar I or bipolar II mood disorder is preceded by cyclothymia, which usually begins in adolescence or early adulthood (Jamison 1996).

Mixed Bipolar States

About 40%–50% of patients with bipolar disorder experience depressive and manic symptoms at the same time (Freeman and McElroy 1999). Manic symptoms in mixed states are usually dys-

---

TABLE 1–12. **DSM-IV-TR criteria for cyclothymic disorder**

A. For at least 2 years, the presence of numerous periods with hypomanic symptoms and numerous periods with depressive symptoms that do not meet criteria for a Major Depressive Episode.   **Note:** In children and adolescents, the duration must be at least 1 year.

B. During the above 2-year period (1 year in children and adolescents), the person has not been without the symptoms in Criterion A for more than 2 months at a time.

C. No Major Depressive Episode, Manic Episode, or Mixed Episode has been present during the first 2 years of the disturbance.

   Note: After the initial 2 years (1 year in children and adolescents) of Cyclothymic Disorder, there may be superimposed Manic or Mixed Episodes (in which case both Bipolar I Disorder and Cyclothymic Disorder may be diagnosed) or Major Depressive Episodes (in which case both Bipolar II Disorder and Cyclothymic Disorder may be diagnosed).

D. The symptoms in Criterion A are not better accounted for by Schizoaffective Disorder and are not superimposed on Schizophrenia, Schizophreniform Disorder, Delusional Disorder, or Psychotic Disorder Not Otherwise Specified.

E. The symptoms are not due to the direct physiological effects of a substance (e.g., a drug of abuse, a medication) or a general medical condition (e.g., hyperthyroidism).

F. The symptoms cause clinically significant distress or impairment in social, occupational, or other important areas of functioning.

---

phoric, taking the form of irritability, anxiety, or dysphoric over-stimulation rather than elation. Such states can be difficult to distinguish from ultradian cycling (discussed in "Rapid Cycling"), in which moods change so rapidly that they seem to blend into each other, and patients with rapid cycling are more likely than other individuals with bipolar disorder to experience mixed states. Subtle mixed states may consist of depression with racing thoughts, decreased need for sleep or preservation of sexual interest, or mania with suicidal and homicidal thoughts. Both conditions probably represent deterioration of a more organized mood disorder—a deterioration associated, at least in some cases, with chronic use of anti-depressants—and the treatments for mixed states and rapid-cycling bipolar disorder are similar.

Rapid Cycling

Having been recognized by Kraepelin at the beginning of the twentieth century, rapid cycling was first described as a specific entity by Dunner and Fieve in 1974. In DSM-IV-TR, rapid cycling is a specifier that refers to a bipolar I or bipolar II mood disorder in which four or more episodes of depression and/or mania or hypomania occur per year, with either 2 weeks of normal mood between episodes or a switch directly from one pole to the other with no intervening period of normal mood. The prevalence of rapid cycling ranges from 12% to 20% among patients with bipolar disorder who are not selected for a high rate of cycling (Baldessarini et al. 2000).

Patients who experienced a switch from one pole to the other within 24 hours were found in one study to be more likely than other patients with rapid cycling to have at least four affective episodes each year during 4 years of follow-up (Maj et al. 1995). However, only a small minority of patients with rapid cycling consistently experience more than four distinct affective episodes per year during prolonged observation (Baldessarini et al. 2000). For many others, mood is chaotic rather than truly cyclical. In either case, even though each episode is shorter in rapid-cycling bipolar disorder than in non-rapid-cycling bipolar disorder, patients with rapid cycling are ill more of the time and have greater morbidity and suicide risk compared with other bipolar disorder patients (Baldessarini et al. 2000).

Rapid cycling is more common among women and among patients with bipolar II disorder; women make up 70%–90% of patients with rapid cycling (Baldessarini et al. 2000). Rapid cycling may be the most common bipolar phenotype among younger patients (Geller and Cook 2000). Additional risk factors for rapid cycling include more years of illness; exposure to antidepressants;

right hemisphere disease; mental retardation; and use of alcohol and stimulants (Baldessarini et al. 2000). Rapid cycling is more likely to occur after an episode of mania or hypomania than after depression. One possible implication of this observation is that reducing manic and hypomanic recurrences may reduce the risk of rapid cycling.

Like other types of bipolar disorder, rapid cycling exists in many forms. Maj et al. (1999) found high rates of interrater reliability for each of four overlapping but different definitions of rapid cycling: the DSM-IV definition, a definition that did not include the duration criterion for affective episodes, and two definitions that did not include the duration criterion and that included either a requirement of at least one direct switch from one pole to the other or a requirement of at least 8 weeks of continuously symptomatic illness during the reference year. These groups differed in response to lithium prophylaxis and in proportions of female patients and patients with bipolar II disorder. Because rapid-cycling subtypes have different courses and treatment responses, studies that do not distinguish between them are likely to produce conflicting results. This may be especially true of studies focusing on the association between rapid cycling and antidepressant use.

One malignant form of rapid cycling is ultradian cycling, in which patients experience multiple, unpredictable recurrences of bipolar depression, dysphoric hypomania, mixed depressive and hypomanic symptoms, and a psychotic energized state, with fleeting euthymia between episodes or an abrupt switch from one pole to the other. A chaos theory model can be used to describe these apparently random mood swings (Kilzieh and Akiskal 1999), which Akiskal (1991) called a "protracted pseudounipolar mixed state," one that fluctuates considerably in intensity and symptoms and can be mistaken for borderline personality disorder or agitated depression.

Like classic rapid cycling, ultradian cycling may be preceded by one or more hypomanic episodes (Post et al. 1990). Mixed states can be difficult to distinguish from ultradian cycling, in which moods alter so quickly that they appear to blend into each other, and mixed states occur more frequently in patients with both rapid cycling and ultradian cycling. Ultradian cycling seems to be even more refractory to treatment than classic rapid cycling (Post et al. 1990).

Rapid and ultradian cycling are probably not separate illnesses but rather phases in the evolution of bipolar disorder—phases at one extreme of a continuum of mood destabilization (Kilzieh and Akiskal 1999; Maj et al. 1995) that may last years but may not be permanent (Kilzieh and Akiskal 1999). This hypothesis is supported by family studies showing that rapid cycling does not breed true in the same way that bipolar II disorder does. For example, the prevalence of rapid cycling as well as of major affective disorders overall was the same among relatives of 29 patients with rapid cycling and relatives of 166 patients with non-rapid-cycling bipolar disorder (Nurnberger et al. 1988). Similarly, a careful study using family history RDC demonstrated that among families of patients with rapid cycling, the prevalence of rapid cycling, bipolar disorder, or unipolar depression was not different from that among families of patients without rapid cycling (Lish et al. 1993).

Masked and Subsyndromal Bipolar Disorder

When features listed in Tables 1–4 and 1–5 are obvious, the diagnosis of a bipolar mood disorder is straightforward. However, brief mood swings with mixed symptoms that wax and wane rather than clearly remit and recur can be more difficult to identify. In one study, for example, more than one-third of patients with bipolar disorder were thought to have unipolar depression even though they had already experienced a first episode of mania or hypomania (Ghaemi and Gaughan 2000). Hypomania presenting not as elation but as anxiety attacks, insomnia, difficulty concentrating, irritability, dysphoria, agitation, impulsivity, or interpersonal sensitivity can easily be mistaken for an anxiety disorder or a personality disorder. Bipolar depression with mixed dysphoric hypomanic symptoms such as anxiety, restlessness, and agitation may be confused with agitated unipolar depression. When mania is associated with a formal thought disorder and with bizarre hallucinations, some bipolar psychoses can be confused with excited schizophreniform psychoses.

Subclinical and masked forms of bipolar disorder range from agitated psychoses to temperamental dysregulation of mood. Hyperthymia, which was originally described by J. Delay in 1946, is a chronic pattern of elevated mood that is less obvious than hypomania. Hyperthymic individuals are expansive, dynamic, joyful, and optimistic and have a robust sense of well-being, a decreased need for sleep, decreased appetites, increased energy, increased creativity, and a family history of bipolar disorder. Although their social and occupational functioning are not necessarily impaired, hyperthymic people are prone to more blatant episodes of hypomania and depression, and their underlying emotional pressure may alienate others. Some investigators consider hyperthymia the premorbid personality style of bipolar disorder (Feline 1993).

Subaffective hypomania may be manifested by such personality traits and displays as arrogance, pushiness, irritability, impatience, insensitivity, talkativeness, emotional intensity, interpersonal hypersensitivity, temper tantrums, promiscuity, restlessness, and unpredictability. Never at a loss for a cutting repartee or an excuse, the person may be at the forefront of new movements and groups, only to lose interest after getting everyone else involved. Mixtures of subsyndromal mania and depression are frequently present, as exemplified by wild jokes with a dark or cynical edge, self-destructive thrill-seeking, or suicidal humor. Individuals with bipolar disorder who are chronically high-strung, moody, exhibitionistic, grandiose, hypersensitive, overreactive, and unstable often are thought to have dramatizing personality disorders such as borderline or narcissistic personality disorder. If they seek excitement through stealing or are habitually aggressive, they may appear to have an antisocial personality disorder. Indeed, a number of diagnostic criteria for borderline personality disorder—unstable, intense relationships; affective instability; inappropriate, intense anger; impulsivity; and recurrent suicidal behavior, for example—are also typical of bipolar mood disorders.

In one study, hysteria or sociopathy had previously been diagnosed in two-thirds of patients with cyclothymia (Akiskal et al. 1977). In another study, 22% of 23 patients with bipolar mood disorders met criteria for a personality disorder (Carpenter et al. 1995). High rates of narcissistic pathology have been noted among people with bipolar mood disorders (Grubb 1997), possibly reflecting subsyndromal grandiosity as well as a chronic attempt to bolster self-esteem that is undermined by feelings of helplessness to control an unpredictable mood. Patients may also attempt to achieve a sense of control over unstable mood and impulsivity by becoming purposefully self-destructive, impulsive, or thrill seeking. A desire to feel that abnormal moods are really under one's control can also lead to use of substances such as cocaine that further destabilize moods. Making the distinction between borderline and narcissistic personality disorders and chronic bipolar disorders therefore can be challenging.

Seasonal Affective Disorder

Many people living in climates in which there are marked seasonal differences in the length of the day have seasonal changes in mood, sleep, and energy (Hellekson 1989). There are also seasonal variations in most mood disorders. For example, unipolar depression is more likely to recur in the spring, whereas bipolar depression is more likely to recur in the fall and mania is more likely to recur during the summer (Barbini et al. 1995). Contrary to popular wisdom, the time of greatest risk of suicide is not during the Christmas holidays but during May and June, probably because patients are more energized during the spring (Hellekson 1989). The seasonal peak in the incidence of suicide is independent of latitude, but the amplitude of the peak is greatest where there is the greatest seasonal variation in light (Hellekson 1989). Hospital admissions for unipolar depression peak in the spring, whereas admissions for mania peak in the summer (Hellekson 1989). The observations that seasonal variations in mood disorders in the Southern Hemisphere are the reverse of those in the Northern Hemisphere (e.g., more admissions for mania during the winter) and that the pattern of seasonal affective disorder (SAD) in the Southern Hemisphere is opposite that in the Northern Hemisphere support the hypothesis that these changes are dependent on variations in available daylight (Hellekson 1989).

SAD was defined by Norman Rosenthal and associates (Hellekson 1989) as a condition that meets criteria for an RDC major affective disorder in which major depression occurs during the fall or winter for at least 2 consecutive years, with remission in the spring or summer. For a diagnosis of SAD to be made, depressive episodes cannot be associated with seasonal stressors, and no other Axis I diagnoses can be present. DSM-IV-TR criteria for the seasonal pattern specifier (Table 1–13), which are derived from the criteria developed by Rosenthal et al. (Hellekson 1989), include provisos that hypomania as well as remission of depression may occur during the summer and that seasonal depressive episodes should substantially outnumber nonseasonal episodes. In DSM-IV-TR, a seasonal pattern is not considered a separate diagnosis but rather a course modifier of MDD with recurrent depression, bipolar I disorder, or bipolar II disorder. The well-described pattern of winter depression and summer euthymia or hypomania is reversed in the Southern Hemisphere (Hellekson 1989). In the Northern Hemisphere, reverse SAD, in which patients become depressed in the summer, seems to be related to seasonal changes in temperature and humidity rather than to changes in light (Hellekson 1989).

SAD occurs more frequently in women than in men, and the female-to-male ratio is greater than for nonseasonal MDD (Hellekson 1989). SAD occurs in children as well as adults (Hellekson 1989). A survey of centers specializing in the treatment of SAD found the most common symptoms during depressive episodes to be sadness, irritability, anxiety, decreased activity, increased appetite with carbohydrate craving, increased weight, increased sleep, daytime drowsiness, work and interpersonal problems, and menstrual difficulties (Hellekson 1989). Symptoms began in November in Washington, D.C., and in late August in Alaska, a finding that supports the role of shortening of the day as precipitant of winter depression. The mean duration of depressive symptoms across centers was

TABLE 1–13. **DSM-IV-TR criteria for seasonal pattern specifier**

Specify if:

With Seasonal Pattern (can be applied to the pattern of Major Depressive Episodes in Bipolar I Disorder, Bipolar II Disorder, or Major Depressive Disorder, Recurrent)

A. There has been a regular temporal relationship between the onset of Major Depressive Episodes in Bipolar I or Bipolar II Disorder or Major Depressive Disorder, Recurrent, and a particular time of the year (e.g., regular appearance of the Major Depressive Episode in the fall or winter).

Note: Do not include cases in which there is an obvious effect of seasonal-related psychosocial stressors (e.g., regularly being unemployed every winter).

B. Full remissions (or a change from depression to mania or hypomania) also occur at a characteristic time of the year (e.g., depression disappears in the spring).

C. In the last 2 years, two Major Depressive Episodes have occurred that demonstrate the temporal seasonal relationships defined in Criteria A and B, and no nonseasonal Major Depressive Episodes have occurred during that same period.

D. Seasonal Major Depressive Episodes (as described above) substantially outnumber the nonseasonal Major Depressive Episodes that may have occurred over the individual's lifetime.

about 5–6 months. More than half the patients had a family history of affective disorder, and many had a family history of SAD.

In some samples, the majority of patients with SAD have summer hypomania and therefore meet criteria for bipolar II disorder; in other samples, the incidence of hypomania is low (Hellekson 1989). Some of the discrepancy may be a function of the frequency with which increased energy, decreased sleep, and related experiences during the summer are viewed as hypomania or simply relief of depression, perhaps with some rebound of mood. More data are needed to determine how frequently SAD is a bipolar subtype and how frequently it is unipolar. There is greater agreement that atypical depressive symptoms, especially hypersomnia and carbohydrate craving, are more common than typical symptoms in the winter depressions of SAD (Hellekson 1989).

Cycloid Psychoses

The concept of cycloid psychosis dates back at least a century in the European literature. In 1893, Magnan described a recurrent condition characterized by the sudden onset of fluctuating psychotic symptomatology, which he called *bouffée délirante*. In 1928, Kleist coined the term *zykloide Psychosen*. The cycloid psychoses are a group of disorders that may represent an interaction between a propensity for psychosis and bipolar dimensions of rapid onset, frequent recurrence, abrupt and complete interepisode recovery, and strong affective coloring but not mania or hypomania. In addition to affective lability, prominent features include confusion, perplexity, and polymorphic psychosis. Three subtypes of cycloid psychoses have been described (von Trostorff and Leonhard 1990). Motility psychosis resembles catatonia in that it is characterized by periods of excitation and stupor, but it does not involve abnormal content or form of thought. Anxiety–happiness psychosis alternates between fear of impending doom or the end of the world and a transcendent sense of having a special mission to save or destroy the world. Confusion psychosis is manifested by agitated or inhibited thought manifested by excited incoherence or perplexed thought blocking. Features of these subtypes often accompany each other or appear in pure form.

It is not yet clear whether cycloid psychoses are atypical bipolar subtypes or whether they should be classified with brief psychotic disorder, schizoaffective disorder, schizophreniform disorder, or other acute primary psychoses. However, differences have emerged between cycloid psychoses and other psychotic illnesses. For example, patients with cycloid psychosis have more visual hallucinations and "delusional mood" but have a better outcome than do patients with schizoaffective disorder (Maj 1988). Even after years of recurrent illness, patients with cycloid psychosis do not have the same ventricular enlargement that is seen in imaging studies of patients with schizophrenia and mood disorders (Hoffler et al. 1997). Cycloid psychoses have been associated with different patterns of the P300 auditory evoked potential than either schizophrenia or bipolar disorder (Strik et al. 1997). The long-term course of cycloid psychoses generally involves less deterioration than either bipolar disorder or schizophrenia (Pfuhlmann 1998).

The 1-year incidence for first psychiatric admission for cycloid psychosis is 5 per 100,000 for women and 3.5 per 100,000 for men; the lifetime prevalence is less than 1% or approximately half of that for schizophrenia (Lindvall et al. 1993). A significant number of cases of postpartum psychosis meet criteria for cycloid psychoses, especially motility psychosis (Pfuhlmann 1998). Bipolar disorder may be diagnosed more frequently in American women with postpartum psychosis, whereas cycloid psychoses are diagnosed more frequently in European women with this presentation, because most American psychiatrists are not familiar with cycloid psychoses.

Neuroleptics alone or in combination with lithium have been reported to be effective acutely for single episodes of cycloid psychosis (Perris 1988). Reports of responses to the newer atypical antipsychotic drugs have not been published. In a number of studies, lithium and carbamazepine (Maj 1984) have reduced the number of recurrences, although it is not clear whether mood stabilizers are effective acutely. ECT has been reported to produce rapid improvement in patients with cycloid psychosis refractory to treatment with medications (Perris 1988). Further exploration of the therapeutic as well as the phenomenological similarities and differences between cycloid psychoses and bipolar disorder may lead to descriptions of more specific subtypes of syndromes in which psychosis interacts with dysregulation of mood, behavior, and thought.

■ SECONDARY MOOD DISORDERS

In some circles, the term *secondary mood disorder* is used to indicate a mood disorder having another cause—for example, a medical illness or a substance. To other experts, a secondary mood disorder is a mood disorder that occurs in the context of another disorder, such as schizophrenia or an anxiety disorder, with etiology not necessarily being implied. DSM-IV-TR implies causality with the terms *mood disorder due to a general medical condition* (mood disorder caused by a medical or surgical illness; see Table 1–14) and *substance-induced mood disorder* (mood disorder caused by a medication or a psychoactive substance; see Table 1–15) ("Drugs That Cause Psychiatric Symptoms" 1993). Affective symptoms that are clearly caused by another condition respond more poorly to treatment than do primary mood disorders.

The other meaning of *secondary mood disorder* has been addressed in two ways in DSM-IV-TR. Although it is permissible to make a diagnosis of a mood disorder in a patient with another Axis I disorder such as schizophrenia, chronic affective symptoms that occur exclusively during the course of a psychotic disorder such as schizophrenia and that do not meet criteria for an independent mood disorder are not given a separate diagnosis of a depressive disorder. In this conceptualization, the affective symptoms are a component of the psychotic illness, and regarding them as such avoids implying meaningless comorbidity. In actual practice, however, treatment of the primary disorder by itself may not resolve the affective symptoms.

■ MOOD DISORDERS IN CHILDREN AND ADOLESCENTS

When it was thought that a mature superego was necessary to develop depression or mania (which was considered a defense against depression), childhood depression was thought to be very rare. As a result, DSM-I did not include psychiatric disorders of children, and DSM-II included only behavioral disorders of children. However, it is now known that depression can be diagnosed in children as young as 3 years. Consequently, DSM-III and DSM-III-R criteria for juvenile mood disorders were similar to those for adult mood disorders, except that irritability could substitute for depressed mood, failure to maintain expected weight gain could substitute for weight loss,

TABLE 1–14. **Some medical conditions that can cause manic or depressive syndromes**

Neurological disease
Parkinson's disease
Huntington's disease
Traumatic brain injury
Stroke
Dementias
Multiple sclerosis

Metabolic disease
Electrolyte disturbances
Renal failure
Vitamin deficiencies or excesses
Acute intermittent porphyria
Wilson's disease
Presence of environmental toxins or heavy metals

Gastrointestinal disease
Irritable bowel syndrome
Chronic pancreatitis
Crohn's disease
Cirrhosis
Hepatic encephalopathy

Endocrine disorders
Hypothyroidism
Hyperthyroidism
Cushing's disease
Addison's disease
Diabetes mellitus
Parathyroid dysfunction

Cardiovascular disease and surgery
Myocardial infarction
Angina
Coronary artery bypass surgery
Cardiomyopathies

Pulmonary disease
Chronic obstructive pulmonary disease
Sleep apnea
Reactive airway disease

Malignancies and hematologic disease
Pancreatic carcinoma
Brain tumors
Paraneoplastic effects of lung cancers
Anemias

Autoimmune disease
Systemic lupus erythematosus
Fibromyalgia
Rheumatoid arthritis

decreased school performance could substitute for decreased occupational function, and loss of interest in friends and play could substitute for loss of interest or pleasure. Symptom duration for a diagnosis of dysthymia in children and adolescents was established as 1 year, as opposed to the required duration of 2 years in adults. These criteria are not been substantially different in DSM-IV-TR.

TABLE 1–15. **Some substances that can cause mania or depression**

Drug	Reactions	Comments
Acyclovir	Psychosis, depression	At high doses
β-Adrenergic blockers	Depression, confusion, mania	At usual doses, including ophthalmologic use
Alcohol	Depression, withdrawal, mania	
Amantadine	Psychosis, mania	More frequent in elderly patients
Amphetamine-like drugs	Psychosis, mania, anxiety, withdrawal, depression	
Anabolic steroids	Mania, depression, psychosis	
Anticonvulsants	Depression, mania	Usually occur when doses or blood levels are high
Antidepressants	Mania; anxiety; abulia with SSRIs	Mania to hypomania in 0.5%–10% of patients
Asparaginase	Depression, paranoia	May occur frequently
Baclofen	Psychosis, mania, depression	Sometimes with treatment and at high doses, but usually with sudden withdrawal
Barbiturates	Depression, excitement	Especially in children and elderly patients
Benzodiazepines	Depression, psychosis, mania	During treatment and withdrawal
Bromocriptine	Mania, psychosis, depression	Not dose related; may persist for weeks after drug therapy is stopped
Bupropion	Mania, psychosis, agitation	Drug can aggravate schizophrenia
Buspirone	Mania, panic attack	In a few patients
Captopril	Mania, anxiety, psychosis	Especially in depressed patients
Carbamazepine	See Anticonvulsants	
Chloroquine	Psychosis, mania	Several reports

TABLE 1–15. **Some substances that can cause mania or depression** *(continued)*

Drug	Reactions	Comments
Clonidine	Depression	May resolve with continued use
Contraceptives, oral	Depression	In 15% in 1 study
Corticosteroids	Mania, depression, psychosis	Especially at high doses or on withdrawal
Cyclobenzaprine	Mania, psychosis	Several reports
Cycloserine	Anxiety, depression, psychosis	Common
Cyclosporine	Psychosis, mania	Each in 1 patient
Dapsone	Psychosis, mania, depression	Several reports, even at low doses
DEET	Mania, psychosis	With excessive or prolonged use
Digitalis glycosides	Psychosis, depression	Especially when doses or blood levels are high
Diltiazem	Depression, suicidal thoughts	8 cases
Disopyramide	Psychosis, depression	Within 24–48 hours of starting therapy
Disulfiram	Depression, psychosis	Not related to alcohol reactions
Enalapril	Depression, psychosis	2 reports
Ethionamide	Depression, psychosis	Multiple reports
Etretinate	Severe depression	
Fenfluramine	See Amphetamine-like drugs	
L-Glutamine	Grandiosity, hyperactivity	In 2 men
Histamine H_2 receptor antagonists	Psychosis, depression, mania	Usually at high doses, more often in elderly patients, more often with renal dysfunction
HMG-CoA reductase inhibitors	Depression	Several cases; may be rare

TABLE 1–15. **Some substances that can cause mania or depression** *(continued)*

Drug	Reactions	Comments
Interferon-α	Delirium, psychosis, depression, suicidal thoughts, mania	Common adverse effects; depression may be treated with SSRIs
Isocarboxazid	See Monoamine oxidase inhibitors	Mania and psychosis in 2 patients during withdrawal
Isoniazid	Depression, psychosis	Several reports
Isosorbide	Psychosis, depression	In 1 elderly woman on 2 occasions
Isotretinoin	Depression	Several reports
Levodopa	Depression, hypomania, psychosis	More common in elderly patients or with prolonged use
Loxapine	Mania	In 1 man
Mefloquine	Psychosis, depression	Several reports
Methyldopa	Depression, psychosis	Several reports
Metoclopramide	Mania, severe depression, crying	Several reports
Metrizamide	Psychosis, depression	May be prolonged
Metronidazole	Depression, crying, psychosis	2 cases with oral use
Monoamine oxidase inhibitors	Mania, psychosis	
Nalidixic acid	Depression	Rare
Narcotics	Euphoria, dysphoria, depression, psychosis	Usually at high doses
Nifedipine	Irritability, depression	Several reports
Nonsteroidal anti-inflammatory drugs	Psychosis, depression	Not reported with all drugs in this class
Norfloxacin	Depression	
Ofloxacin	Depression, mania	Single reports of each
Penicillin G procaine	See Procaine derivatives	
Pergolide	Psychosis, depression	On withdrawal

TABLE 1–15. **Some substances that can cause mania or depression** *(continued)*

Drug	Reactions	Comments
Phenelzine	See Monoamine oxidase inhibitors	
Phentermine	See Amphetamine-like drugs	
Phenylephrine	Depression, psychosis	Overuse of nasal spray; single report with oral use
Phenylpropanolamine	See Amphetamine-like drugs	
Phenytoin	See Anticonvulsants	
Prazosin	Psychosis, depression	In 4 patients; 2 had renal failure
Procaine derivatives	Psychosis, depression, anxiety	Many reports, especially with penicillin G procaine
Procarbazine	Mania	In 2 children
Propafenone	Psychosis, mania	Several reports
Pseudoephedrine	Psychosis, mania	Reported at usual doses in children and with overuse in 1 adult
Quinacrine	Mania, psychosis	More common at high doses
Reserpine	Depression	Common at doses >0.5 mg/day
Selegiline	See Monoamine oxidase inhibitors	
Sulfonamides	Depression, euphoria	Several reports
Theophylline	Mania, depression	Usually with high serum concentrations
Thiazides	Depression, suicidal ideation	In several patients after weeks to months of use
Thyroid hormones	Mania, depression, psychosis	Initial doses in susceptible patients

TABLE 1–15. **Some substances that can cause mania or depression** *(continued)*

Drug	Reactions	Comments
Tranylcypromine	See Monoamine oxidase inhibitors	Hypomania or mania in up to 10% of depressed patients
Trimethoprim-sulfamethoxazole	Psychosis, depression	Several reports
Valproic acid	See Anticonvulsants	
Vinblastine	Depression	
Vincristine	Depression	
Zidovudine	Mania, psychosis	2 cases

Note. DEET=diethyltoluamide; HMG-CoA=3-hydroxy-3-methylglutaryl coenzyme A; SSRI=selective serotonin reuptake inhibitor.

MDD occurs in as many as 18% of preadolescents, with no sex differences (Kashani and Nair 1995). The prevalence of MDD has been reported to be 4.7% among 14- to 16-year-olds (Kashani and Nair 1995). By this age, depression is more common among girls than boys. In nonclinical samples, up to one-third of adolescents reported some depressive symptoms (Kashani and Nair 1995). Major depression in adolescents is associated with substance abuse and antisocial behavior, both of which sometimes obscure the affective diagnosis. The lifetime prevalence of bipolar disorder was 0.6% among 150 adolescents who were not psychiatrically referred (Kashani and Nair 1995). Many cases of bipolar disorder in younger patients might be overlooked because mania has not yet appeared or because, when it is present, it is manifested by anxiety, irritability, and attentional and behavioral syndromes that mask the mood disorder.

Because of continued disagreement about the nature of juvenile mood disorders, estimates of prevalence and incidence vary. When the Schedule for Affective Disorders and Schizophrenia for School-Aged Children was administered to 1,710 adolescents ages 14–18 years, almost 30% were found to have at least one current depressive symptom, the most common symptoms being depressed mood, disturbed sleep, problems thinking, and anhedonia (Roberts et al. 1995). However, only 2.6% of the sample met full criteria for a current diagnosis of a mood disorder. In contrast to adults in other studies, adolescents in this study who had experienced two episodes of major depression had different symptoms during each episode. Compared with adult mood disorders, childhood mood disorders have been found to have more familial loading, and when children from depressed families become depressed, the depression occurs earlier than the depression that occurs in children from families that are not depressed (ages 12–13 years vs. ages 16–17 years) (Geller et al. 1996). These kinds of findings suggest that inherited factors may be more important in juvenile mood disorders, as in other early-onset medical disorders. Mood disorders in younger patients, as in adults, present a definite risk of suicide, especially when they are complicated by substance use; the cumulative prevalence of suicide attempts among adolescents is as high as 3% (Shaffer et al. 1996). On the other hand, early intervention in childhood and adolescent mood disorders improves long-term outcome.

One area of ongoing investigation is the presentation of bipolar disorder in children and adolescents. Compared with adult bipolar disorder, juvenile bipolar disorder is characterized by less elation and more irritability, dysphoria, psychosis, schizophreniform symptoms, hyperactivity, mixed mania, rapid cycling, chronicity, and familial loading (Geller et al. 1995). An important question that clinicians often face is whether a first episode of major depression in a younger patient is more likely than a first episode in an adult to be the initial presentation of a bipolar mood disorder (i.e., to be followed by the later development of mania or hypomania) (Akiskal 1995; Kashani and Nair 1995). When conservative criteria are used, between 5% and 15% of cases of major depression in adults are bipolar, compared with at least 20% of cases among adolescents and 32% of cases among children less than 11 years old (Geller et al. 1996). Features that juvenile major depressive episodes share with bipolar disorder include an early age at onset, equal numbers of males and females affected, mood lability, a high rate of recurrence, prominent irritability and explosive anger suggestive of mixed bipolar episodes, and a relatively poor response to antidepressants (Akiskal 1995). In addition, juvenile major depressive episodes are often associated with cyclothymic or hyperthymic temperaments (Akiskal 1995).

The diagnostic challenge implied by these kinds of observations is to identify those juvenile patients with major depressive episodes who are at greater risk of a bipolar outcome and who might have better ultimate responses to mood-stabilizing treatments than to antidepressants. Some features of major depressive episodes in younger patients have been found to increase the likelihood of eventual occurrence of mania (Akiskal 1995; Strober and Carlson 1982) (see Table 1–16). Although no predictive studies exist regarding the prognostic validity of these features, their occurrence in younger patients with bipolar disorder is reason for caution in treating juvenile major depression. One of these factors in particular warrants additional discussion. As we noted in "Bipolar Subtypes," hypomania that occurs only when antidepressants are being taken is excluded in DSM-IV-TR as a diagnostic criterion for bipolar disorder in adults, because not all patients with this experience become manic spontaneously. However, several small studies involving depressed adolescents and children have indicated a very high rate of spontaneous mania or hypomania among juvenile patients who experienced antidepressant-induced hypomania (Akiskal 1995).

Difficulty recognizing juvenile bipolar disorder accounts for the finding in one report that half the children who fulfilled diagnostic criteria for mania had received a different diagnosis first (Kashani and Nair 1995). A particularly controversial area of diagnostic confusion concerns attention-deficit/hyperactivity disorder (ADHD). Some reports suggest a familial link between juvenile bipolar disorder and ADHD, and these conditions are frequently diagnosed together. For example, in a study in which 28% of 270 psychiatric inpatients ages 5–18 years who were given the Schedule for Affective Disorders and Schizophrenia for School-Aged Children met criteria for ADHD, 36% of the patients with ADHD met criteria for nonpsychotic depression, 8% met criteria for an affective psy-

TABLE 1–16. **Features associated with a bipolar outcome in juvenile major depression**

Early onset
Acute onset
Highly recurrent depression
Appearing less depressed than the patient feels
Preservation of energy and interest despite severe depression
Psychotic symptoms, especially hallucinations
Significant psychomotor slowing
Family history of bipolar disorder
Any mood disorder in three consecutive generations
Antidepressant-induced hypomania

chosis, and 22% met criteria for bipolar disorder (Butler et al. 1995); there was no follow-up to determine how many of the depressed patients developed mania.

Clinical experience also suggests that ADHD and bipolar disorder are often diagnosed in the same patient, but it is not clear whether this means that the two disorders are frequently comorbid or that the symptoms of the two disorders overlap, so that patients who meet criteria for one condition will regularly also meet criteria for the other (Butler et al. 1995). The latter point is illustrated in Table 1–17 (Kashani and Nair 1995).

Most patients with bipolar disorder meet virtually all criteria for ADHD, but despite the symptomatic overlap, patients with ADHD do not meet all criteria for bipolar disorder (Geller et al. 1998). For example, elation, depression, suicidality, hypersexuality, decreased need for sleep, hypersomnia, grandiosity, psychosis, ultradian cycling, and rapid, pressured speech are much more characteristic of childhood bipolar disorder than of ADHD (Geller et al. 1998; Kashani and Nair 1995), although stimulant toxicity can of course induce psychosis. Racing and tangential thinking may be difficult to differentiate from the kind of talkativeness that is encountered in patients with ADHD, but an increased content of thought, especially with multiple coexisting complex ideas and plans, is more suggestive of bipolar disorder than of ADHD. Irrita-

TABLE 1–17. **Common features of attention-deficit/
hyperactivity disorder (ADHD) and
juvenile bipolar disorder**

ADHD	Bipolar disorder[a]
Mood lability, temper outbursts	Mood lability, temper outbursts
Failure to give close attention to detail	(Racing thoughts, impulsivity)
Difficulty sustaining attention	Racing thoughts
Failure to listen when spoken to directly	Self-involvement
Failure to follow through	(Impulsivity, distractibility, tangential thinking, changeable direction of effort driven by mood swings)
Difficulty organizing tasks and activities	(Disorganization, changeable focus of attention, impulsivity)
Loses things necessary for tasks	(Distractibility, impulsivity)
Easily distracted	Distractibility
Forgetfulness in daily activities	(Fluctuating interest and motivation)
Fidgets or squirms	(Increased levels of activity)
Leaves seat when remaining seated is expected	Increased energy
Excessive running about or climbing	Increased activity
Difficulty playing quietly	Increased energy and activity
Often on the go or as if driven by a motor	Increased energy and activity
Excessive talking	Pressure of speech
Blurting out of answers before questions have been completed	Racing thoughts
Difficulty awaiting turn	(Impulsivity, increased energy)
Interrupts or intrudes on others	(Impulsivity, grandiose self-centeredness)

[a]DSM-IV-TR features (and, in parentheses, features that are not formal diagnostic criteria) of bipolar disorder that could be mistaken for ADHD.

bility, fighting, and thrill seeking can occur in both disorders, but attacks of rage that provoke prolonged organized attacks on others in response to threats to self-esteem and attempts to control the patient are more common in bipolar disorder, as is the kind of grandiosity that leads to fighting multiple opponents, fearlessness in the face of overwhelming odds, and jumping from heights with the belief that one cannot be hurt and a response of hilarity to being injured. Heavy familial affective loading appears to be more common in bipolar disorder. Finally, the index of suspicion for bipolar disorder should probably be higher in tertiary care centers, given that uncomplicated ADHD is usually treated successfully in the offices of pediatricians and family physicians and by psychiatrists who consult to schools, and patients who see specialists generally present with more complex illnesses.

A study involving 140 boys ages 6–17 years with diagnoses of ADHD attempted to address the question of symptomatic overlap by rediagnosing patients' conditions after specific symptoms of ADHD had been subtracted (Milberger et al. 1995). Seventy-nine percent of the patients still met criteria for MDD, 56% met criteria for bipolar disorder, and 75% met criteria for generalized anxiety disorder. One interpretation is that these disorders share a sufficient number of characteristics similar to those of ADHD (and each other) to result in patients meeting criteria for more than one of them at the same time. Another is that a diagnosis of ADHD is not very specific in adolescents with mood and anxiety disorders.

A positive response to stimulants is often interpreted as evidence in favor of a diagnosis of ADHD. However, the positive effect of stimulants on attention is not specific to ADHD. Depressed patients with slowed thinking may show improvement of attention with stimulant use, and some manic patients have been noted to experience calming and behavioral slowing in response to stimulants (Max et al. 1995). Although no controlled studies have addressed this issue, adolescent and young adult patients are encountered in practice who were apparently treated successfully with stimulants or antidepressants for ADHD, only to develop dysphoric manic symptoms such as increasing irritability, anxiety, impulsivity, thrill seeking, grandiose defiance, mood swings, and psychosis with continued treatment. It is impossible to know whether long-term administration of stimulants eventually destabilized mood in these patients with bipolar disorder misdiagnosed as ADHD or whether the adverse outcome represented the natural progression of bipolar disorder.

Deciding whether to institute treatment for bipolar disorder, ADHD, or both in situations in which a juvenile patient's condition might qualify for either diagnosis is not easy. Stimulants probably have fewer adverse effects and are easier to monitor than mood-stabilizing medications, and they may improve attention in patients with bipolar disorder. However, prolonged use may induce mania and/or rapid cycling, which is more difficult to treat than less complicated forms of bipolar disorder. With the exceptions of clonidine and cholinesterase inhibitors such as donepezil, medications used in bipolar disorder have never been thought to be helpful in ADHD, but they do not pose any special risks in patients with ADHD. It would therefore seem prudent to initiate treatment with a mood-stabilizing medication in unclear cases. If the increased rate of apparent co-occurrence of bipolar disorder and ADHD is evidence of comorbidity as well as of symptom overlap, a distinct subpopulation will have both disorders. In this case, ADHD symptoms should persist after treatment of the mood disorder, at which time the need for additional treatment of ADHD can be assessed, assuming that the ADHD symptoms are not side effects of antimanic drugs. If nonpharmacological treatments are not effective for the residual attentional symptoms, a cholinesterase inhibitor might be considered before a stimulant, an antidepressant such as bupropion, or another dopaminergic agent.

■ MOOD DISORDERS AND CREATIVITY

An association between mood disorders, especially bipolar mood disorders, and creativity has been noted for some time. Reviews of the histories of prominent artists and writers suggest that Honoré de Balzac, Lord Byron, F. Scott Fitzgerald (and his wife, Zelda),

Ernest Hemingway, Randall Jarrell, Charles Lamb, Robert Lowell, Theodore Roethke, Delmore Schwartz, Anne Sexton, and Virginia Woolf had bipolar disorder (Jamison 1996). Andreasen (1987) found that 80% of 30 writers at a creative writing workshop had experienced at least one affective episode, and 43% had a history of hypomania or mania; the relatives of these writers also had increased rates of both mood disorders and creativity. In a study of 20 award-winning European writers, painters, and sculptors, two-thirds had recurrent cyclothymia or hypomania, and half had experienced depressive episodes (Jamison 1996).

Jamison found that 38% of distinguished British writers and visual artists had been treated for a mood disorder (Jamison 1996). In her book *Touched With Fire: Manic-Depressive Illness and the Artistic Temperament,* Jamison (1993) reviewed the personal histories of well-known artists and writers with mood disorders, many of them bipolar. Other biographical studies, as well as studies involving living artists, demonstrate that compared with the general population, individuals who are successful in the arts are up to 18 times as likely to commit suicide, 8–10 times as likely to have major depressive episodes, and 10–20 times as likely to have a bipolar mood disorder (Jamison 1996).

The apparent link between mood disorders and creativity has yet to be examined systematically. One possibility is that the elevated energy and expansive thinking of manic and hypomanic individuals may contribute to increased frequency of ideas, and an increased rate and content of thought may result in unique ways of synthesizing ideas (Jamison 1996). High levels of energy and of mental and physical activity and a decreased need for sleep can enhance productivity, but activity in bipolar disorder is usually uneven and at times impulsive and self-defeating, and periods of energetic hyperactivity are often interrupted by episodes of depressive torpor. Another possibility is that ordinary situations are experienced so intensely by people with mood disorders that these situations can be communicated more powerfully to others, although an active mood disorder is at least as likely to make the artist feel overwhelmed and disorganized by minor events. It is also conceivable that artistic people with mood disorders are more likely to put themselves in adverse situations that result in the kinds of experiences that can be successfully represented in their art. Equally compelling is the possibility that genes that influence creativity are linked to genes that increase the risk of bipolar disorder.

It is important to note, lest mood disorders, and bipolar illness in particular, be romanticized as necessary for artistic success, that most people with mood disorders are not particularly creative (Jamison 1996), and many highly creative people do not have mood disorders. In creative people with mood disorders, there is no evidence that active illness actually improves creativity or that successful treatment hinders artistic careers. If anything, treatment of mood disorders improves productivity (Jamison 1993) and can make an artist's work more comprehensible and organized.

■ CATEGORICAL VERSUS DIMENSIONAL DIAGNOSES

The DSM-III/DSM-IV/DSM-IV-TR approach to diagnosis has facilitated the description of more homogeneous populations so that course and treatment outcomes can be better studied. Symptom specifiers such as *with atypical features* and course modifiers such as *seasonal pattern* represent a preliminary attempt to define subtypes of mood disorders that might have different responses to treatment. However, no categorical mood disorder diagnosis is as uniform or as useful clinically as is suggested in the diagnostic manual (Brown et al. 1994). Some affective disorders are mild, and others are severe. Some people with bipolar disorder have many manic episodes, and some do not. Some depressed individuals who never experience a hint of mania have recurrences of depression more frequently than do patients with bipolar depression. Some patients with bipolar depression become psychotic, as do some patients with unipolar depression. Some depressed people are very aggressive or suicidal, and some are not. Some people who are prone to depression have had traumatic experiences early in life, some have had families who misunderstood or did not care about them, and some have had highly supportive families. Some kinds of depression start early in life without any particular precipitant, some begin only after a stressful event, and some appear for the first time in later years. Some mood disorders are associated with substantial character pathology, and some are not. Some are accompanied by medical and psychiatric comorbidity, and some are not.

Mood disorders are diverse physiologically as well as phenomenologically. Within a given DSM-IV-TR diagnosis (e.g., MDD), some subtypes are accompanied by one of the laboratory markers discussed in the next chapter, some by a different marker, and some by no known marker. Some patients have obvious familial transmission of a mood disorder that has similar manifestations in most family members, and some have sporadic illnesses. Some manic episodes respond to lithium, some to an anticonvulsant, and some only to combinations of drugs. Even within the same individual, the presentation and treatment response of affective episodes may vary from one episode to the next.

Within categorical constraints, there are thus many dimensions of abnormal mood, and the expression of a given type of mood disorder will depend on the net interaction between these factors (Figure 1–2). This is not to say that every depressed person is different from every other depressed person; rather, more varieties of depression, and more treatment options, exist in real life than are listed in the textbooks. For example, a classification system based on cluster analysis that included severity as a diagnostic dimension was more useful than DSM diagnosis in predicting impairment of mental and physical health in a primary care setting (Nease et al. 1999). As more knowledge accumulates about the importance of specific dimensions of depression, it may become possible to make dimensional as well as categorical diagnoses that suggest more specific treatment options.

■ COMORBIDITY

Mood disorders are frequently comorbid with other psychiatric and medical conditions, especially anxiety, substance-related, eating,

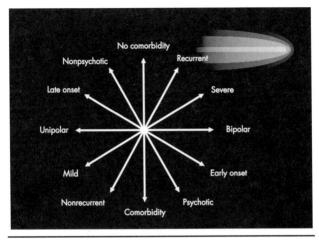

FIGURE 1–2. **Dimensions of mood disorders.**

somatoform, and personality disorders and chronic medical illnesses (Weissman et al. 1996). In one study of this issue, the Department of Veterans Affairs database was used to compare records of 11,701 medically ill patients with those of 9,039 psychiatric patients (Moos and Mertens 1996). As many as 60% of patients with mood disorders treated in mental health settings had a comorbid psychiatric diagnosis, as did 30% of mood disorder patients treated in medical settings. Eighty percent of the psychiatric patients had comorbid medical conditions.

Medical Illness

The prevalence of major depressive episodes among patients with malignancies has been reported to be around 50% among those with pancreatic cancer, 22%–40% among those with cancer of the oropharynx, 10%–32% among patients with breast cancer, 13%–25% among those with colon cancer, and 23%, 17%, and 11% among patients with gynecological cancer, lymphoma, and gastric carcinoma, respectively (McDaniel et al. 1995). Depression was found in 16% of bone marrow transplant recipients (Fann and Tucker 1995). Major depression occurs at increased rates in patients with myocardial infarction, ventricular arrhythmias, or congestive heart failure (Franco-Bronson 1996), whereas major depression has been found to increase the risk of coronary heart disease and to increase mortality after myocardial infarction (Barefoot and Schroll 1996).

Hypothyroidism is common in depressed patients, especially in those with treatment-refractory mood disorders and rapid-cycling bipolar disorder. Much of the hypothyroidism that occurs in depressed patients is caused by thyroiditis, which suggests a link between susceptibility loci for major depression and thyroiditis. There appears to be a similar link between migraine headaches and MDD, possibly because both are associated with hyperreactive blood platelets. A subgroup analysis of the Baltimore Epidemiologic Catchment Area study findings revealed that the lifetime risk of self-reported migraine headaches was increased 3.14 times in current major depression (Swartz et al. 2000). Additional medical conditions frequently associated with depression include irritable bowel syndrome, fibromyalgia, chronic fatigue syndrome, AIDS, renal failure, and autoimmune disease.

A number of neurological illnesses are also associated with an increased risk of mood disorders (Fann and Tucker 1995). Between 8% and 75% of patients with cerebrovascular accidents develop major depression; in one study, stroke patients with depression had an eightfold risk of mortality compared with matched stroke patients who were not depressed (Morris et al. 1993). Stroke location appears to have a marked effect on the prevalence of associated depression: left prefrontal and basal ganglia strokes more frequently result in depressive disorders than do right hemisphere lesions. Conversely, right hemisphere lesions are often associated with development of secondary mania. Cerebrovascular and degenerative disease on the left side of the brain causes late-onset depression, and disease on the right side of the brain is often associated with late-onset mania. Depression is the most frequent psychiatric complication of Parkinson's disease, possibly because of the participation of the basal ganglia in mood regulation (Klassen et al. 1995).

About 50% of patients with Alzheimer's disease meet criteria for major depression or dysthymia, whereas 2%–3.8% of Alzheimer's disease patients develop mania (Fann and Tucker 1995). Despite the fact that the pattern of dementia is cortical in Alzheimer's disease and subcortical in the dementia syndrome of depression, it can be impossible to distinguish one from the other clinically, and depression can aggravate the dementia of Alzheimer's disease. The interaction between depression and dementia was discussed in the section on "Masked Depression." The incidence of depression is also increased in temporal lobe epilepsy, AIDS, Huntington's disease, traumatic brain injury, spinal cord injury, and multiple sclerosis; and AIDS and traumatic brain injury can also present as mania (Fann and Tucker 1995).

Anxiety Disorders

Anxiety occurs as a prominent nonspecific symptom in as many as 70% of depressed outpatients. In addition, comorbidity of mood and anxiety disorders has been found consistently in large studies (Weissman et al. 1996). The National Institute of Mental Health Collaborative Study on the Psychobiology of Depression found that 32% of depressed patients had phobias, 31% had panic attacks, and 11% had obsessions or compulsions (Glass et al. 1989). Conversely, major depressive episodes have been reported in 8%–39% of patients with generalized anxiety disorder, 50%–90% of patients with panic disorder, 35%–70% of patients with social phobia, and 33% of patients with obsessive-compulsive disorder (Gorman and Coplan 1996). Social phobia has been reported in more than 40% of patients with MDD. Bipolar illness is also frequently comorbid with panic disorder and obsessive-compulsive disorder.

There are a number of possible associations between mood and anxiety disorders. For example, anxiety as a signal of hyperactive arousal in response to the perception of danger may be a stage in the development of mood disorders (Figure 1–3), persisting as an

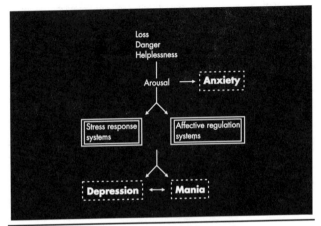

FIGURE 1–3. **Evolution of anxiety and depression.**

enduring symptom of a hyperactive stress response. Many kinds of distress in depressed patients can be referred to as anxiety, and patients may describe arousal and dysphoria as anxiety at one point and depression at another. Some patients cannot tell the difference between anxiety and depression, and some of the items on mood rating scales such as the Ham-D are symptoms of anxiety. Some of the time, anxiety may reflect a separate disorder that occurs at a higher-than-expected rate in depressed patients; this rate may be higher because one disorder lowers the threshold for the expression of the other or because susceptibility to one disorder is linked to susceptibility to the other. Manic overstimulation may be expressed as panic attacks, which can be distinguished from panic disorder by the presence of racing thoughts and a sense of having too much energy. Anxiety in patients with bipolar mood disorders is often an indication of mixed (dysphoric) states.

Alternating emphasis on particular symptoms probably accounts for the observation that a group of patients with depressive disorders followed prospectively might be given new diagnoses of anxiety disorders, whereas patients with initial diagnoses of anxiety disorders may receive later diagnoses of mood disorders. In some instances, the predominance of one or the other symptom may represent a prodromal phase of a mood disorder in which both anxiety and depression are important symptoms. The extent to which one disorder is emphasized over the other (e.g., depression with secondary anxiety or anxiety with secondary depression) may be more a matter of features that strike the examiner or the patient at a particular moment than of the nature of the illness.

In addition to their comorbidity, depression, mania, and anxiety as dimensions of affective experience overlap and interact with each other in complex ways. Anxiety in depressed patients increases severity, chronicity, and impairment associated with depression and makes depression more refractory to treatment; anxiety also increases the risk of suicide in depressed patients, perhaps because it is a marker of higher levels of arousal. Depressed people who are anxious have a greater number of anxious relatives, and they also have more familial loading for depression (Clayton et al. 1991).

Substance Use Disorders

Major mood disorders have high rates of comorbidity with use of many substances, especially alcohol (Weissman et al. 1996). Alcohol abuse or dependence occurs in 50% of patients with unipolar depression, 60% of patients with bipolar I disorder, and 50% of patients with bipolar II disorder. The Epidemiologic Catchment Area study found that about one-third of individuals with mood disorders had a comorbid substance use disorder (McDowell and Clodfelter 2001). Comorbid alcoholism worsens the course of both unipolar depression and bipolar disorder. Conversely, abstinence improves the response of the mood disorder to treatment (Hasin et al. 1996).

The prevalence of depression among individuals with substance dependence is higher among active drinkers, which is not surprising because alcohol, as with a number of other substances, can cause depression (Table 1–15). In one study, the prevalence of depression among alcohol-dependent patients decreased from 67%

when they were actively drinking to 13% after detoxification (Davidson 1995). Such findings, as well as studies demonstrating reduced rates of response to antidepressants during active alcohol use, have led to the clinical practice of deferring treatment for depression until substance use has been curtailed. However, recent work with substance-dependent adolescents suggests that the presence of depression interferes with patients' ability to engage in treatment for the substance use disorder (Rao et al. 2000) and that antidepressant therapy that improves depressive symptoms may reduce alcohol consumption in nonabstinent depressed alcoholic individuals (McGrath et al. 1996). These observations may support the concurrent treatment of depression and substance use in some patients. It may be productive in some cases to treat depression before the patient becomes fully abstinent.

Use of sedatives by manic patients to tone down dysphoric overstimulation is readily understandable. The reason some patients with bipolar mood disorders use stimulants (especially cocaine) to induce mania would be obvious if the mania were pleasurable, but substance-induced mania is frequently dysphoric. By purposely making themselves manic, some of these patients may be attempting to achieve the illusion of mastery over fluctuations in mood that otherwise feel completely unpredictable and uncontrollable. Patients with mood disorders who are treated acutely with neuroleptics may note blunting of the rewarding properties of cocaine, but chronic neuroleptic therapy, which is common treatment for patients who have been hospitalized for bipolar mood disorders, may enhance the euphoric effects of cocaine by leading to postsynaptic dopamine receptor supersensitivity in reward centers.

Schizophrenia

Major depressive episodes occur in 25%–50% of cases of schizophrenia. The traditional belief that most of these episodes are "postpsychotic" and involve reactions to awareness of having a severe illness is contradicted by the finding that half the depressive episodes occurring during the course of schizophrenia develop in the midst of an acute psychotic episode, but the affective component may become apparent only after the psychosis resolves (Dubovsky and Thomas 1992). Fears that administration of antidepressants may aggravate schizophrenia have been contradicted by observations that in all but the most acute psychotic exacerbations, treatment of concomitant depression improves the prognosis of schizophrenia (Dubovsky and Thomas 1992).

Personality Disorders

Between 30% and 70% of depressed patients with unipolar or bipolar disorder receive a concurrent diagnosis of a personality disorder, usually in Cluster B (i.e., borderline, narcissistic, histrionic, or antisocial personality disorder) (Corruble et al. 1996). At the same time, 95% of personality disorder patients who commit suicide have a comorbid Axis I diagnosis, usually a mood disorder (Isometsa et al. 1996). It was noted previously that personality disorders may be diagnosed frequently in association with mood disorders because pathological defenses mobilized to deal with an increased pressure of mood mimic character pathology. Thase and colleagues (Thase 1996) found that when they reinterviewed depressed patients after successful treatment, the rate of personality disorder was half the rate before treatment. Assessment of the role of personality disorders is further complicated by a tendency of clinicians to attribute to a personality disorder the failure of depressed patients to respond as expected (Thase 1996).

There are a number of additional possible explanations for the association between mood and personality disorders (Thase 1996). One possibility is that certain personality traits or disorders may predispose to mood disorders. For example, an overly dependent patient might be more vulnerable to depression in response to loss of an important source of support, and a perfectionistic person would be more likely to become depressed in response to not performing perfectly (see Chapter 2). It is also possible that chronic mood disorders may skew experience in ways that lead to the development of personality disorders, as when grandiosity, impulsivity, expansiveness, and a high threshold for experiencing stimulation (because baseline levels of emotional arousal are so high in bipolar mood disorder) become integrated into a patient's habitual behavioral repertoire, leading to histrionic and narcissistic traits and chronic sensation-seeking. Finally, vulnerability to depression and to personality disorders may be inherited or acquired together, or common etiological factors may lead to both mood and personality disorders.

Compared with mood disorder patients without personality disorders, patients with mood disorders who have comorbid personality disorders have more overall symptomatology, experience worse social adjustment, and are less responsive to interpersonal psychotherapy, antidepressants, and ECT (Thase 1996). However, cognitive-behavioral therapy has been reported to be equally effective in depressed patients with and without personality disorders (Thase 1996). The negative impact of an Axis II diagnosis on the outcome of a mood disorder may be directly attributable to the personality disorder, or it may simply be an indication of a more pervasive and therefore severe mood disorder.

In clinical practice, apparent comorbid personality disorders that actually reflect exaggeration of pathological character traits often are not as problematic when the mood disorder responds to treatment. On the other hand, personality traits and behaviors such as self-destructive motivations, negative therapeutic reactions, and attachment to an identity as a depressed person can lead to noncompliance, turning of treatments against the clinician, and other behaviors that interfere with a positive response to treatment. If these issues are not addressed, treatment of the mood disorder is not likely to be successful.

■ REFERENCES

Akiskal HS: Chronic depression. Bull Menninger Clin 55:156–171, 1991

Akiskal HS: Developmental pathways to bipolarity: are juvenile-onset depressions pre-bipolar? J Am Acad Child Adolesc Psychiatry 34:754–763, 1995

Akiskal HS: The prevalent clinical spectrum of bipolar disorders: beyond DSM-IV. J Clin Psychopharmacol 16:4S–14S, 1996

Akiskal HS, Djenderedjian AM, Rosenthal RH, et al: Cyclothymic disorder: validating criteria for inclusion in the bipolar affective group. Am J Psychiatry 134:1227–1233, 1977

American Psychiatric Association: Diagnostic and Statistical Manual: Mental Disorders. Washington, DC, American Psychiatric Association, 1952

American Psychiatric Association: Diagnostic and Statistical Manual of Mental Disorders, 2nd Edition. Washington, DC, American Psychiatric Association, 1968

American Psychiatric Association: Diagnostic and Statistical Manual of Mental Disorders, 3rd Edition. Washington, DC, American Psychiatric Association, 1980

American Psychiatric Association: Diagnostic and Statistical Manual of Mental Disorders, 3rd Edition, Revised. Washington, DC, American Psychiatric Association, 1987

American Psychiatric Association: Diagnostic and Statistical Manual of Mental Disorders, 4th Edition. Washington, DC, American Psychiatric Association, 1994

American Psychiatric Association: Diagnostic and Statistical Manual of Mental Disorders, 4th Edition, Text Revision. Washington, DC, American Psychiatric Association, 2000

Andreasen NC: Creativity and mental illness: prevalence rates in writers and their first-degree relatives. Am J Psychiatry 144:1288–1292, 1987

Angst J: Epidémiologie du spectre bipolaire. Encephale 21 (Spec No 6):37–42, 1995

Angst J, Hochstrassen B: Recurrent brief depression: the Zurich Study. J Clin Psychiatry 55 (suppl):3–9, 1994

Angst J, Wicki W: The Zurich Study, XI: is dysthymia a separate form of depression? Results of the Zurich Cohort Study. Eur Arch Psychiatry Clin Neurosci 240:349–354, 1991

Angst J, Merikangas K, Scheidegger P, et al: Recurrent brief depression: a new subtype of affective disorder. J Affect Disord 19:87–98, 1990

Baldessarini RJ, Tondo L, Floris G, et al: Effects of rapid cycling on response to lithium maintenance treatment in 360 bipolar I and II disorder patients. J Affect Disord 61:13–22, 2000

Barbini B, Di-Molfetta D, Gasperini M, et al: Seasonal concordance of recurrence in mood disorder patients. Eur Psychiatry 10:171–174, 1995

Barefoot JC, Schroll M: Symptoms of depression, acute myocardial infarction, and total mortality in a community sample. Circulation 93:1976–1980, 1996

Beck CT: A meta-analysis of the relationship between postpartum depression and infant temperament. Nurs Res 45:225–230, 1996

Belsher G, Costello CG: Relapse after recovery from unipolar depression: a critical review. Psychol Bull 104:84–96, 1988

Blazer DG, Koenig HG: Mood disorders, in Textbook of Geriatric Psychiatry. Edited by Busse EW, Blazer DG. Washington, DC, American Psychiatric Press, 1996, pp 235–264

Brown S-L, Steinberg RL, van Praag HM: The pathogenesis of depression: reconsideration of neurotransmitter data, in Handbook of Depression and Anxiety. Edited by den Boer JA, Sitsen JMA. New York, Marcel Dekker, 1994, pp 317–347

Butler SF, Arredondo DE, McCloskey V: Affective comorbidity in children and adolescents with attention deficit hyperactivity disorder. Ann Clin Psychiatry 7:51–55, 1995

Carpenter D, Clarkin JF, Glick ID, et al: Personality pathology among married adults with bipolar disorder. J Affect Disord 34:269–274, 1995

Cassano GB, Akiskal HS, Perugi G, et al: The importance of measures of affective temperaments in genetic studies of mood disorders. J Psychiatr Res 26:257–268, 1992

Clayton PJ, Grove WM, Coryell W, et al: Follow-up and family study of anxious depression. Am J Psychiatry 148:1512–1517, 1991

Corruble E, Ginestet D, Guelfi JD: Comorbidity of personality disorders and unipolar major depression: a review. J Affect Disord 37:157–170, 1996

Coryell W: Psychotic depression. J Clin Psychiatry 57 (suppl 3):27–31, 1996

Davidson KM: Diagnosis of depression in alcohol dependence: changes in prevalence with drinking status. Br J Psychiatry 166:199–204, 1995

Dell DL, Stewart DE: Menopause and mood: is depression linked with hormone changes? Postgrad Med 108:39–43, 2000

Drugs that cause psychiatric symptoms. Med Lett Drugs Ther 35:65–70, 1993

Dubovsky SL: Mind-Body Deceptions. New York, WW Norton, 1997

Dubovsky SL, Thomas M: Psychotic depression: advances in conceptualization and treatment. Hospital and Community Psychiatry 43:1189–1198, 1992

Dunner DL, Fieve RR: Clinical factors in lithium carbonate prophylaxis failure. Arch Gen Psychiatry 30:229–233, 1974

Fann JR, Tucker GJ: Mood disorders in patients with general medical condition. Current Opinion in Psychiatry 8:13–18, 1995

Feline A: Les hyperthymies. Encephale 19:103–107, 1993

First NB, Donovan S, Frances A: Nosology of chronic mood disorders. Psychiatr Clin North Am 19:29–39, 1996

Frances AJ: An introduction to dysthymia. Psychiatric Annals 23:607–608, 1993

Franco-Bronson K: The management of treatment-resistant depression in the medically ill. Psychiatr Clin North Am 19:329–350, 1996

Freeman MP, McElroy SL: Clinical picture and etiologic models of mixed states. Psychiatr Clin North Am 22:535–546, 1999

Geller B, Cook EH Jr: Ultradian rapid cycling in prepubertal and early adolescent bipolarity is not in transmission disequilibrium with val/met COMT alleles. Biol Psychiatry 47:605–609, 2000

Geller B, Sun K, Zimerman B, et al: Complex and rapid-cycling in bipolar children and adolescents: a preliminary study. J Affect Disord 34:259–268, 1995

Geller B, Todd RD, Luby J, et al: Treatment-resistant depression in children and adolescents. Psychiatr Clin North Am 19:253–267, 1996

Geller B, Williams M, Zimerman B, et al: Prepubertal and early adolescent bipolarity differentiate from ADHD by manic symptoms, grandiose delusions, ultra-rapid or ultradian cycling. J Affect Disord 51:81–91, 1998

Ghaemi SN, Gaughan S: Novel anticonvulsants: a new generation of mood stabilizers? Harv Rev Psychiatry 8:1–7, 2000

Glass DR, Pilkonis PA, Leber WR, et al: National Institute of Mental Health Treatment of Depression Collaborative Research Program. Arch Gen Psychiatry 46:971–982, 1989

Goodwin FK, Jamison KR: Manic Depressive Illness. New York, Oxford University Press, 1991

Gorman JM, Coplan JD: Comorbidity of depression and panic disorder. J Clin Psychiatry 57 (suppl 10):34–41, 1996

Grubb D: Three Bipolar Women: The Boundary Between Bipolar Disorders and Disorders of the Self. New York, Brunner/Mazel, 1997

Gwirtsman HE, Blehar MC, McCullough JP, et al: Standardized assessment of dysthymia: report of a National Institute of Mental Health conference. Psychopharmacol Bull 33:3–11, 1997

Hasin DS, Tsai W-Y, Endicott J, et al: Five-year course of major depression: effects of comorbid alcoholism. J Affect Disord 41:63–70, 1996

Hellekson C: Phenomenology of seasonal affective disorder: an Alaskan perspective, in Seasonal Affective Disorders and Phototherapy. Edited by Rosenthal NE, Blehar MC. New York, Guilford, 1989, pp 33–43

Hirschfeld RMA: Guidelines for the long-term treatment of depression. J Clin Psychiatry 55 (suppl):61–69, 1994

Hirschfeld RMA, Klerman GL, Lavori P: Premorbid personality assessments of first onset of major depression. Arch Gen Psychiatry 46:345–350, 1989

Hoffler J, Braunig P, Kruger S, et al: Morphology according to cranial computed tomography of first-episode cycloid psychosis and its long-term-course: differences compared to schizophrenia. Acta Psychiatr Scand 96:184–187, 1997

Isometsa ET, Henriksson MM, Heikkinen ME: Suicide among subjects with personality disorders. Am J Psychiatry 153:667–673, 1996

Jamison KR: Touched With Fire: Manic-Depressive Illness and the Artistic Temperament. New York, Free Press, 1993

Jamison KR: Manic-depressive illness, genes, and creativity, in Genetics and Mental Illness: Evolving Issues for Research and Society. Edited by Hall LL. New York, Plenum, 1996, pp 111–132

Kashani JH, Nair J: Affective/Mood disorders, in Diagnosis and Psychopharmacology of Childhood and Adolescent Disorders, 2nd Edition. Edited by Weiner JM. New York, Wiley, 1995, pp 229–263

Keller MB: Dysthymia in clinical practice: course, outcome and impact on the community. Acta Psychiatr Scand Suppl 383:24–34, 1994

Keller MB, Hanks DL, Klein DN: Summary of the DSM-IV mood disorders field trial and issue overview. Psychiatr Clin North Am 19:1–27, 1996

Kendler KS: The diagnostic validity of melancholic major depression in a population-based sample of female twins. Arch Gen Psychiatry 54:299–304, 1997

Kilzieh N, Akiskal HS: Rapid-cycling bipolar disorder: an overview of research and clinical experience. Psychiatr Clin North Am 22:585–607, 1999

Klassen T, Verhey FRJ, Rozendaal N: Treatment of depression in Parkinson's disease: a meta-analysis. J Neuropsychiatry Clin Neurosci 7:281–286, 1995

Klein DN, Kocsis JH, McCullough JP, et al: Symptomatology in dysthymic and major depressive disorder. Psychiatr Clin North Am 19:41–53, 1996

Kleist K: Ueber zykloide, paranoide und epileptoide Psychosen und über die Frage der Degenerationspsychosen. Schweizer Archives der Neurologie und Psychiatrie 23:3–37, 1928

Kocsis JH: DSM-IV "major depression": are more stringent criteria needed? Depression 1:24–28, 1993

Kraepelin E: Manic-Depressive Insanity and Paranoia. Translated by Barclay RM. Edinburgh, Livingstone, 1921

Lepine J, Pelissolo A, Weiller E, et al: Recurrent brief depression: clinical and epidemiological issues. Psychopathology 28 (suppl 1):86–94, 1995

Lindvall M, Axelsson R, Ohman R: Incidence of cycloid psychosis: a clinical study of first-admission psychotic patients. Eur Arch Psychiatry Clin Neurosci 242:197–202, 1993

Lish JD, Gyulai L, Resnick SM, et al: A family history study of rapid-cycling bipolar disorder. Psychiatry Res 48:37–46, 1993

Magnan V: Leçons cliniques, 2nd Edition. Paris, Bataille, 1893

Maj M: Effectiveness of lithium prophylaxis in schizoaffective psychoses: application of a polydiagnostic approach. Acta Psychiatr Scand 70:228–234, 1984

Maj M: Clinical course and outcome of cycloid psychotic disorder: a three-year prospective study. Acta Psychiatr Scand 78:182–187, 1988

Maj M, Magliano L, Pirozzi R, et al: Is rapid cycling a valid subtype of bipolar disorder? Eur Neuropsychopharmacol 5:228–232, 1995

Maj M, Pirozzi R, Formicola AM, et al: Reliability and validity of four alternative definitions of rapid-cycling bipolar disorder. Am J Psychiatry 156:1421–1424, 1999

Max JE, Richards L, Hamdan-Allen G: Case study: antimanic effectiveness of dextroamphetamine in a brain-injured adolescent. J Am Acad Child Adolesc Psychiatry 34:472–476, 1995

McDaniel JS, Musselman DL, Proter MR: Depression in patients with cancer. Arch Gen Psychiatry 52:89–99, 1995

McDowell DM, Clodfelter RC: Depression and substance abuse: considerations of etiology, comorbidity, evaluation, and treatment. Psychiatric Annals 31:244–251, 2001

McElroy SL, Keck PE Jr, Pope HG Jr, et al: Clinical and research implications of the diagnosis of dysphoric or mixed mania or hypomania. Am J Psychiatry 149:1633–1644, 1992

McGrath PJ, Nunes EV, Stewart JW, et al: Imipramine treatment of alcoholics with primary depression: a placebo controlled clinical trial. Arch Gen Psychiatry 53:232–240, 1996

Milberger S, Biederman J, Faraone SV, et al: Attention deficit hyperactivity disorder and comorbid disorder: issues of overlapping symptoms. Am J Psychiatry 152:1793–1799, 1995

Mitchell PB, Wilhelm K, Parker G, et al: The clinical features of bipolar depression: a comparison with matched major depressive disorder patients. J Clin Psychiatry 62:212–216, 2001

Moos RH, Mertens JR: Patterns of diagnoses, comorbidities, and treatment in late-middle-aged and older affective disorder patients: comparison of mental health and medical sectors. J Am Geriatr Soc 44:682–688, 1996

Morris PLP, Robinson RG, Samuels J: Depression, introversion and mortality following stroke. Aust N Z J Psychiatry 27:443–449, 1993

Nease DE, Volk RJ, Cass AR: Investigation of a severity-based classification of mood and anxiety symptoms in primary care patients. J Am Board Fam Pract 12:21–31, 1999

Nurnberger J, Guroff JJ, Hannovit J, et al: A family study of rapid-cycling bipolar illness. J Affect Disord 15:87–91, 1988

Perris C: The concept of cycloid psychotic disorder. Psychiatr Dev 6:37–56, 1988

Pfuhlmann B: Das Konzept der zykloiden Psychosen. Fortschr Neurol Psychiatr 66:1–9, 1998

Post RM, Kramlinger KG, Altshuler LL, et al: Treatment of rapid cycling bipolar illness. Psychopharmacol Bull 26:37–47, 1990

Rao U, Daley SE, Hammen C: Relationship between depression and substance use disorders in adolescent women during the transition to adulthood. J Am Acad Child Adolesc Psychiatry 39:215–222, 2000

Reynolds CF III, Hoch CC: Differential diagnosis of depressive pseudodementia and primary degenerative dementia. Psychiatric Annals 17:743–748, 1987

Roberts RE, Lewinsohn PM, Seeley JR: Symptoms of DSM-III-R major depression in adolescence: evidence from an epidemiological survey. J Am Acad Child Adolesc Psychiatry 34:1608–1617, 1995

Rohde A, Manerous A: Schizoaffective disorders with and without onset in the puerperium. Eur Arch Psychiatry Clin Neurosci 242:27–33, 1992

Scott J: Chronic depression. Br J Psychiatry 153:287–297, 1988

Shaffer D, Gould MS, Fisher P, et al: Psychiatric diagnosis in child and adolescent suicide. Arch Gen Psychiatry 53:339–348, 1996

Shea MT, Hirschfeld RM: A chronic mood disorder and depressive personality. Psychiatr Clin North Am 19:103–120, 1996

Soares JC, Mann JJ: The anatomy of mood disorders—review of structural neuroimaging studies. Biol Psychiatry 41:86–106, 1997

Strik WK, Fallgatter AJ, Stoeber G, et al: Specific P300 features in patients with cycloid psychosis. Acta Psychiatr Scand 95:67–72, 1997

Strober M, Carlson G: Bipolar illness in adolescents with major depression. Arch Gen Psychiatry 39:549–555, 1982

Swartz KL, Pratt LA, Armenian HK, et al: Mental disorders and the incidence of migraine headaches in a community sample: results from the Baltimore Epidemiologic Catchment area follow-up study. Arch Gen Psychiatry 57:945–950, 2000

Thase ME: Relapse and recurrence in unipolar major depression: short-term and long-term approaches. J Clin Psychiatry 51 (suppl):51–57, 1990

Thase ME: Long-term treatments of recurrent depressive disorders. J Clin Psychiatry 53 (suppl):32–44, 1992

Thase ME: The role of Axis II comorbidity in the management of patients with treatment-resistant depression. Psychiatr Clin North Am 19:287–309, 1996

Tsuang D, Coryell W: An 8-year follow-up of patients with DSM-III-R psychotic depression, schizoaffective disorder and schizophrenia. Am J Psychiatry 150:1182–1188, 1993

von Trostorff S, Leonhard K: Catamnesis of endogenous psychoses according to the differential diagnostic method of Karl Leonhard. Psychopathology 23:259–262, 1990

Weissman MM, Bland RC, Canino GJ, et al: Cross-national epidemiology of major depression and bipolar disorder. JAMA 276:293–299, 1996

Winokur G: Manic-depressive disease (bipolar): is it autonomous? Psychopathology 28 (suppl 1):51–58, 1995

2

ETIOLOGY OF MOOD DISORDERS

Mood disorders are truly biopsychosocial disorders, with contributions from all three spheres to etiology and outcome. Etiological factors can be understood on many levels, from the role of inherited and sociological factors to changes in gene expression and cellular functioning. An enormous amount of information has accumulated about the physiology of mood disorders in particular. When interpreting studies of etiological factors in mood disorders, it is important to be aware that there is not likely to be a single cause of even the most rigidly defined mood disorder. As van Praag (1990) pointed out, "Though a lot of biology has been uncovered in mental disorders, most of it seems to be devoid of nosological specificity" (p. 2).

■ INHERITED FACTORS

There is no reason to think that any inborn factor by itself causes mood disorders; such factors interact with experiential and other environmental influences to lead to illness. In addition, the expression of inherited factors is itself complex. One abnormal gene may produce an abnormal protein that contributes to a positive symptom, whereas another gene may fail to make a protein that regulates the emergence of the same symptom. Data in favor of genetic influences in mood disorders suggest that these disorders are oligogenic, reflecting the interaction of multiple gene products.

Family Studies

Careful studies have repeatedly demonstrated that mood disorders
are familial. Relatives of people with mood disorders are consistently two to three times as likely to have mood disorders as are relatives of control subjects (Gershon 1990). If one parent has a
bipolar mood disorder, the risk that a child will have a unipolar or
bipolar mood disorder is around 28%; if both parents have mood
disorders, the risk is two to three times as great (Jamison 1996). Patients with mood disorders also have an increased familial incidence of substance abuse, and patients who are depressed and
anxious have more relatives who are depressed, anxious, or both
(Gorman and Coplan 1996).

Wealth and political affiliation also run in families, but they are
not genetic. One way to begin to identify a genetic contribution is
to compare the concordance of mood disorders in first- and second-
degree relatives of probands with mood disorders. Because first-
degree relatives (parents, children, and siblings) share 50% of their
genomes, whereas only 25% of genes are shared by second-degree
relatives (grandparents, uncles, aunts, nephews, and nieces), a
greater rate of a mood disorder among first-degree relatives of individuals with the same disorder than among second-degree relatives
of these individuals suggests a genetic influence (Tsuang and
Faraone 1996). The expectation of a greater likelihood of mood disorders among first-degree relatives of patients with mood disorders
than among second-degree relatives or control populations has usually been confirmed (Tsuang and Faraone 1996).

Most studies suggest a more prominent familial transmission of
bipolar than of unipolar mood disorders, often with affected relatives in consecutive generations. In addition, the age at symptom
onset is earlier in individuals with bipolar disorder who have
strongly positive family histories. Family members of patients with
bipolar disorder are more likely to have bipolar as well as unipolar
mood disorders themselves than are family members of patients
with unipolar disorders (Jamison 1996). However, the rate of bipolar disorder among the families of patients with unipolar depression

is as much as three to four times the rate among control subjects (Gershon et al. 1982). According to published family studies, first-degree relatives of patients with unipolar depression have a risk of unipolar depression of 5.5%–28.4% and a risk of bipolar disorder of 0.7%–8.1%, and first-degree relatives of probands with bipolar disorder have a 4.1%–14.6% likelihood of having a bipolar disorder themselves and a 5.4%–14% likelihood of having unipolar depression (Gershon et al. 1982; Tsuang and Faraone 1996). Familial overlap has also been found between schizophrenia and mood disorders. As noted in Chapter 1, bipolar II disorder "breeds true"; that is, patients with bipolar II disorder have relatives who are hypomanic but not manic, whereas patients with bipolar I disorder have some relatives who are manic and some who are hypomanic (Jamison 1996).

Twin Studies

Another approach to investigating genetic contributions to mood disorders is to study differences in concordance between monozygotic (identical) and dizygotic (fraternal) twins. Monozygotic twins come from the same egg and have the same genes, whereas dizygotic twins come from different eggs and share 50% of their genes, like any other siblings. A greater concordance rate for a disorder among monozygotic twins than among dizygotic twins suggests a genetic influence because the role of intrauterine and postnatal environments is presumably similar for both kinds of twins (Tsuang and Faraone 1996). Concordance studies (Jamison 1996; Tsuang and Faraone 1996) reliably demonstrate that the overall risk of mood disorders is three times as great among monozygotic than among dizygotic twins of probands with mood disorders. For bipolar disorder, concordance rates average 0.67–1.0 for monozygotic and 0.20 for dizygotic twins. Concordance rates for unipolar depression are generally 0.50 among monozygotic twins and 0.20 among dizygotic twins. The greater difference in concordance rates between monozygotic and dizygotic twins with regard to bipolar disorder may reflect a greater genetic influence in bipolar disorder.

The assumption that identical twins grow up in identical environments may not be entirely accurate. The phase of division of the egg at which two embryos begin to emerge differs in different monozygotic twin pairs, and this has potential implications for later development of the nervous system. Because parents and other close caretakers can usually tell monozygotic twins apart, not all sets of monozygotic twins are exposed to the same interpersonal fields as they grow up. Concordance rates for mood disorders among monozygotic twins reared apart from infancy can help to differentiate genetic influences from potential differences in the postnatal environment. In one study, 8 of 12 monozygotic twins of probands with bipolar mood disorders had bipolar mood disorders themselves, a rate similar to the concordance rate among monozygotic twins of bipolar mood disorder patients reared with their ill twins (Jamison 1996).

Because concordance rates for mood disorders in twin studies are less than 100%, any genetic factors that are present must interact with environmental influences to create the risk for development of the actual disorder (Tsuang and Faraone 1996). Reviews of twin studies suggest that 21%–45% of the variance in the risk of depressive disorders can be attributed to genetic factors and that 55%–75% of the variance can be attributed to environmental factors (Kendler et al. 1993). A substantial amount (60%) of the effect of genetic factors appears to be direct, but 40% seems to reflect genetic factors that increase the likelihood that people will put themselves in situations that lead to depression (e.g., becoming romantically involved with someone who is likely to leave) (Kendler et al. 1993). Of stressful life events, losses seem to be most influential (Kendler et al. 1993).

We mentioned in "Family Studies" that patients with major depression and comorbid anxiety have both anxiety and depression in their families. In addition, Kendler et al. (1992) reported that 1,033 pairs of female twins had increased concordance for both major depression and generalized anxiety disorder, agoraphobia, and social phobia. Kendler et al. (1992, 1993) hypothesized that some common trait predisposing to anxiety and depression may be inherited and that experience determines whether anxiety or depression will predominate clinically.

Adoption Studies

The influence of the environment on the development of mood disorders can also be assessed by examining rates of mood disorders in adoptive and biological families of people who were adopted in infancy. Most of these studies find that adoptees with mood disorders are more likely to have biological than adoptive relatives with mood disorders (Tsuang and Faraone 1996). Adoptive studies suggest that both genetic and adoptive (i.e., environmental) factors are important in determining transmission of unipolar depression and suicide (Tsuang and Faraone 1996). The observation that rates of bipolar disorder in adoptive families of probands with bipolar disorder are no greater than in the general population, whereas rates of bipolar disorder in the biological families of these adoptees are the same as those among individuals with bipolar disorder who were raised with family members having the same illness, suggests that adoptive factors do not play a significant role in bipolar mood disorders (Tsuang and Faraone 1996), although experiences in the adoptive family may influence when and how bipolar disorder is expressed.

Linkage Studies

Less inferential studies of genetic factors examine linkage between mood disorders and specific genetic markers or discrete biological phenotypes such as activity of an enzyme or physiological function (endophenotype). Presumably, a gene or genes influencing development of the mood disorder would be close to the genes for the phenotype or the genetic marker that aggregates with the mood disorder. Linkage studies are most reliable for disorders that have a single dominant gene mode of transmission with complete penetrance, such as Huntington's disease. Unfortunately, the mode of transmission of most mood disorders is oligogenic, and incomplete penetrance and variable expressivity are likely to be the rule (Tsuang and Faraone 1996). Because the familial pattern of some bipolar mood disorders seems more consistent with a dominant mode of transmission, linkage studies involving families with bipolar disorder have been most promising.

Red-green color blindness, a recessive X-linked trait, has been linked to bipolar mood disorders in about one-third of cases studied (Tsuang and Faraone 1996). An X-linked factor near the gene for color blindness would be expected to demonstrate mother-to-son transmission, which is observed in some families with bipolar disorder. Of three linkage studies involving glucose-6-phosphate dehydrogenase (G6PD) deficiency, the gene for which is thought to be close to the gene for color blindness, findings of one supported and findings of another were highly suggestive of linkage of G6PD deficiency to bipolar disorder (Tsuang and Faraone 1996). A study of the F9 DNA marker on the X chromosome suggested linkage to bipolar disorder, but studies of other DNA markers from the same region did not reveal such linkage (Tsuang and Faraone 1996). Results of studies of linkage of bipolar mood disorder to different traits thought to be carried on the X chromosome may not have been more consistent because some bipolar subtypes in some families have X-linkage whereas others do not. Additional reasons for apparently contradictory findings in linkage studies are discussed later in this section.

Attempts to link human leukocyte antigen phenotypes to bipolar mood disorders have generally been unsuccessful (Tsuang and Faraone 1996). The fact that bipolar disorder and thalassemia minor cosegregated in a family seemed to suggest linkage to a gene on the short arm of chromosome 11 close to the HRAS1 locus, because thalassemia minor is caused by a mutation at that locus (Joffe et al. 1986). This possibility was interesting because HRAS may be involved in the translation of experience into changes in neuronal functioning. However, these results have not been replicated. An association between bipolar mood disorder and blood type O, the gene for which is on chromosome 9, was found in one study (Lavori et al. 1984). This finding was also of theoretical interest because the ABO blood type gene is close to the gene for dopamine β-hydroxylase; however, additional studies have rejected the concept of linkage of bipolar disorder to ABO markers (Tsuang and Faraone 1996).

A more specific type of linkage analysis involves restriction fragment length polymorphisms (RFLPs), which are DNA fragments prepared by digestion of chromosomes with restriction endonucleases that break DNA at known nucleotide sequences. Each RFLP contains more than one gene. In a widely publicized RFLP study of bipolar disorder in a large pedigree of Old Order Amish (Egeland et al. 1987), linkage was found to an RFLP on the short arm of chromosome 11 (11p15), another finding of theoretical interest because this locus is close to the gene for tyrosine hydroxylase, the rate-limiting step in the synthesis of norepinephrine. The model derived from this study suggested a penetrance of about 60%; that is, about 60% of subjects with a specific allele of the marker had a diagnosis of bipolar disorder. Unfortunately, additional data from patients who did not have the 11p15 marker but developed bipolar disorder appeared to refute the original findings and actually exclude linkage to chromosome 11p15 (Kelsoe et al. 1989), and European studies of different pedigrees never showed linkage to 11p15 in the first place (Berrettini et al. 1997).

Studies of other loci have yielded equally confusing results. An investigation involving one family suggested linkage of bipolar disorder to the long arm of chromosome 11, but other work rejected this hypothesis (Tsuang and Faraone 1996). Suggestions of linkage of bipolar disorder to markers on chromosome 21q22.3 in a few families were refuted in later research (Vallada et al. 1996). A study of 310 DNA markers covering about 50% of the genome excluded linkage of bipolar I disorder; bipolar II disorder; schizoaffective disorder, bipolar type; and recurrent unipolar depression to all markers except a marker on the centromeric region of chromosome 18 (Berrettini et al. 1997). However, linkage to chromosome 18 was not confirmed in another study involving five families (Maier et al. 1995).

There are a number of possible reasons why genetic markers for bipolar disorder are reported in one study and refuted in another (Berrettini et al. 1997; Tsuang and Faraone 1996). Methodologies used differ substantially, as do diagnostic instruments and even definitions of unipolar and bipolar disorder. Even though bipolar and unipolar mood disorders can run in the same families as a result of assortative mating, they probably have different patterns of familial aggregation, and bipolar II disorder has a different familial pattern than does bipolar I disorder. Yet linkage studies do not distinguish between bipolar I disorder and bipolar II disorder, and many studies group subjects with schizoaffective disorder and even recurrent unipolar depression with bipolar disorder patients so that there will be enough patients to achieve statistically significant findings. If attempts are made to distinguish between unipolar disorder and bipolar disorder in a linkage study, patients with bipolar disorder who have not yet had a manic episode may be counted as unipolar disorder patients, as apparently happened in the Amish study (Egeland et al. 1987). If patients with subsyndromal bipolar mood disorders are counted as unipolar disorder patients, evidence of an association between a particular marker and bipolar disorder will be diluted. Given the oligogenic nature of most mood disorders, it seems likely that positive associations that are found reflect some dimension of the mood disorder (such as recurrence, severity, thought disorder, or psychosis) or a comorbid condition that is subject to genetic influences (such as anxiety, substance use, or attention-deficit/hyperactivity disorder). Additional methodological issues include possible genetic differences between ethnic groups that are lumped together in genetic studies, and flaws in statistical assumptions on which measures of significance are based.

Even it were possible to overcome financial and technical barriers to large, multicenter studies involving homogeneous populations of patients with narrowly defined bipolar or unipolar mood disorders, and more discrete genetic markers could be employed, there are several reasons why contradictory findings are likely to continue to emerge from linkage studies. First, there is no reason to believe that only one inherited factor predisposes to a given mood disorder, no matter how much patients with the disorder resemble one another clinically. Any one of a number of genes could produce abnormal proteins that alter a cascade of physiological events at different points to produce the same end result. Another gene might fail to produce a protein with sufficient activity to keep the abnormal cascade from having an effect. Similarly, entirely different genes might affect different processes, each of which lowers the threshold for expression of the same complex syndrome. The same phenotype therefore could be associated with any one of a number of genotypes. In addition, because individuals with mood disorders tend to marry one other at a greater-than-random rate (assortative mating), members of the same family are likely to have genetically different mood disorders. Conversely, variable expressivity and penetrance can result in patients with the same genotype having phenotypically distinct disorders. Finally, some cases of a mood disorder in a given family may clinically resemble a genetic form of the disorder without there being any genetic contribution at all (phenocopies), whereas spontaneous mutations can result in new cases of a genetic form of mood disorder in the absence of a prominent family history of the disorder.

The implication of these complexities is not that linkage and other genetic studies of mood disorders are invalid but that the genetic component of mood disorders is probably underestimated by the current methodology. Subsequent negative findings in the Amish study do not mean that there is no linkage between bipolar disorder and chromosome 11p15; rather, some cases of bipolar disorder in this population probably do have a genetic contribution at this locus, whereas others do not. Some bipolar disorders probably are X-linked, some are sporadic, and some may have no genetic influence. The degree to which a pathogenic gene is expressed in a particular mood disorder probably depends on interactions of the gene with experience and with other genes. The earlier the onset of the mood disorder, the less time has elapsed for adverse experience to cause it and the greater the importance of genetic factors. Similarly, the greater the incidence of mood disorders in consecutive generations in the family, the more important the genetic influence is likely to be.

■ IMAGING FINDINGS

In view of evidence presented in Chapter 1 that injury to left frontal anterior cortical or subcortical areas causes secondary depression, whereas right-sided lesions in the limbic system, temporobasal areas, basal ganglia, and thalamus induce secondary mania, it is possible that subtle alterations in the structure or function of brain areas that participate in mood regulation could contribute to primary mood disorders. Relevant areas of the brain for this kind of formulation include the prefrontal cortex; subcortical structures such as the basal ganglia, thalamus, and hypothalamus; the brain stem; and white matter pathways connecting these structures to one other and the cerebral cortex (e.g., the limbic-thalamic-cortical circuit and the limbic-striatal-pallidal-thalamic-cortical circuit), and possibly the cerebellum (Soares and Mann 1997). Abnormalities in these areas that could contribute to affective symptoms might be caused by abnormal brain development, vascular injury, aging, or degenerative disease.

A variety of findings have emerged from structural and brain imaging studies involving depressed patients (Soares and Mann 1997). One of the most consistent generalized brain abnormalities in structural imaging studies of unipolar depression has been enlarged lateral ventricles, which are reported most frequently in late-onset major depressive disorder (MDD). Subcortical white matter and periventricular hyperintensities have been noted on magnetic resonance images in older but not younger patients with unipolar depression. Regional abnormalities most consistently reported in unipolar depression have included decreased size of the caudate, putamen, and possibly the cerebellum. The basal ganglia receive input from medial temporal structures that regulate emotion, such as the amygdala and hippocampus, but there has not been any reliable evidence of abnormalities in the amygdala and hippocampus in mood disorders. Reduced frontal lobe volume has been variably reported. Loss of glial and other cells in the hippocampus is reversible after early episodes but becomes irreversible after depression has been present for extended periods.

Imaging studies involving patients with bipolar mood disorders (Geller et al. 1996; Soares and Mann 1997) have found enlarged third ventricles at all ages in adults (and in a small sample of children), as well as the same kinds of subcortical white matter and periventricular hyperintensities and the same loss of glial cells that is seen in older patients with unipolar depression. White matter hyperintensities on magnetic resonance images increase with age in patients with bipolar mood disorders but not in control subjects, suggesting an interaction between aging and diagnosis (Woods et al. 1995). Because the presence of psychotic symptoms may be correlated with enlarged lateral ventricles in depressed patients, and because psychotic features are more frequent in bipolar depression than in unipolar depression, ventricular enlargement in bipolar disorder patients at any age may be linked more closely to psychosis than to bipolarity. However, although enlarged lateral ventricles are more common in major depression with psychotic features, white matter hyperintensities are not (Soares and Mann 1997). In contrast to unipolar depression, no consistent magnetic resonance imaging changes in the frontal lobes have been reported in bipolar mood disorders (Soares and Mann 1997).

Subcortical white matter hyperintensities found in older patients with unipolar depression and bipolar disorder patients of any age may be better markers of cerebrovascular disease than of the mood disorder (Soares and Mann 1997). This could explain why a greater volume of abnormal white matter in bipolar mood disorder patients is correlated with more cognitive impairment (Dupont et al. 1995). A substrate of neurological dysfunction associated with white matter hyperintensities could also account for an increased risk of delirium with electroconvulsive therapy (ECT); extrapyramidal side effects with administration of neuropsychotic medications; chronicity; and overall poor treatment response in patients with this magnetic resonance imaging finding (Dupont et al. 1995; Soares and Mann 1997).

Although some argue that enlarged ventricles and sulci are found more frequently and that the severity of structural brain changes is greater in mood disorders than in schizophrenia, others point out that such findings occur in many psychiatric and medical illnesses, especially mood disorders, schizophrenia, and Alzheimer's disease (Soares and Mann 1997). The most cogent explanation for apparent structural abnormalities in primary mood disorders is that they identify neuroanatomical substrates that can cause secondary mood disorders in older patients and that contribute to dementia syndromes in interaction with a primary mood disorder. In primary mood disorders, neurological factors may lead to treatment resistance and greater cognitive impairment, but there is no evidence that they are etiological in most cases. However, although microvascular disease in particular may contribute to gross brain changes and to pseudodementia, hypercortisolemia (see "Dexamethasone Suppression Test") may be a more important cause of hippocampal damage in patients with chronic mood disorders.

Cerebral Blood Flow Findings

Functional brain imaging with positron emission tomography and single photon emission computed tomography (SPECT) is used to measure regional cerebral blood flow, which is closely related to regional brain metabolism. Positron emission tomography has demonstrated reduced metabolic activity in the frontal lobes (i.e., hypofrontality) in unipolar (Buchsbaum et al. 1997) and bipolar (Gyulai et al. 1997) depression. Antidepressants were found to normalize frontal metabolic activity (Buchsbaum et al. 1997). Asymmetries in cerebral blood flow have also been found in depression, but such findings have been variable.

Most but not all SPECT studies using technetium Tc 99m hexamethylpropyleneamine oxime have demonstrated reduced global cerebral blood flow in depressed patients compared with control subjects, with localized perfusion deficits in frontal, prefrontal, cingulate, temporal, and sometimes parietal and subcortical regions (Bonne et al. 1996). Iofetamine I 123 SPECT in 12 rapid-cycling bipolar disorder patients in manic, depressed, and euthymic states showed greater uptake in the right than in the left anterior temporal lobe in both the depressed and manic phases but not during euthymia, which suggests state-dependent metabolic asymmetry in both poles of abnormal mood (Gyulai et al. 1997). Some functional imaging studies have found hyperactivity of the amygdala, hippocampus, and some temporal structures (Doris et al. 1999).

Neuropathology

Pathological studies of brains of patients with mood disorders are complicated by factors such as sample size, methods of brain fixation, and reliability of diagnoses. However, a few findings have appeared to be reliable (Vawter et al. 2000). For example, loss of glial cells in the left prefrontal cortex has been demonstrated in both bipolar and unipolar mood disorders, whereas decreased size and density of gray matter neurons in the same region was found in MDD. Loss of glial cells and neurons in the hippocampus has been repeatedly noted in mood disorders.

■ ELECTROENCEPHALOGRAPHIC FINDINGS

The same type of cerebral asymmetry has been found in electroencephalographic studies of major depression, with less left frontal activation and greater right frontal activation (as measured by alpha suppression) in major depression (Davidson 1992). Davidson (1992) suggested that reduced left frontal activation is associated with a deficit in approach-related behaviors and that right frontal activation is associated with an increase in withdrawal-related behaviors. The interpretation of electroencephalographic findings is complicated by the fact that depression and anxiety may have additive effects on anterior activation and contradictory effects on parietotemporal electroencephalographic activity (Bruder et al. 1997). Bruder et al. (1997) found less left than right anterior cortical activation in depressed patients with comorbid anxiety disorders, but not in depressed patients without anxiety disorders. In contrast, nonanxious depressed patients had less activation at right posterior sites than at left posterior sites. These patterns could reflect differences in mobilization of the stress response in primarily anxious versus primarily depressed patients. As is true of genetic studies, such findings illustrate the possibility that abnormalities are linked to specific dimensions of the mood disorder rather than to global diagnosis.

■ BIOLOGICAL MARKERS AND TESTS

Clear associations have been established between mood disorders and alterations in biological functioning measurable in the laboratory. Most biological markers are reported more frequently in patients with severe, psychotic, or bipolar mood disorders and in inpatients, who are of course more severely ill. However, few markers have consistently distinguished between bipolar and unipolar mood disorders. Although there has been extensive theorizing on the issue, it is not certain whether well-replicated biological markers reflect a process that is a cause or a result of mood disorders.

Dexamethasone Suppression Test

The dexamethasone suppression test (DST) was initially used to study adrenal cortical activity in mood disorders because hypercortisolemia has repeatedly been observed in depressed patients. In the DST, 1 mg of dexamethasone (a synthetic adrenal steroid) is given in the afternoon to effect feedback inhibition at the level of the pituitary and the hypothalamus of cortisol production by the adrenal cortex, and serum cortisol levels are measured one or more times the following day. Because the assay for cortisol does not read dexamethasone, the level of cortisol the day after dexamethasone administration is a measure of how readily the hypothalamic-pituitary-adrenal-cortical axis can be suppressed. Normally, cortisol levels decrease to 5 μg/dL or less with dexamethasone suppression. Hyperactivity at any point between the hypothalamus and the adrenal cortex can be associated with failure of dexamethasone suppression, demonstrated by cortisol levels >5 μg/dL after administration of dexamethasone (i.e., nonsuppression).

Melancholic major depression is associated with a 40%–50% rate of dexamethasone nonsuppression (Brown et al. 1994). The frequency of nonsuppression is higher (80%–90%) in patients with severe or psychotic unipolar depression, patients with major depression who have made more severe suicide attempts, inpatients, and persons with a family history of affective disorder (Rush et al. 1997). Bipolar depression and mania are associated with the same frequency of dexamethasone nonsuppression as melancholic unipolar depression (Rush et al. 1997). The DST is usually a state variable; DST results convert to normal 1–3 weeks before clinical remission, and reversion to nonsuppression occurs within 1–3 weeks of clinical relapse (Brown et al. 1994; Rush et al. 1997).

The proximate cause of dexamethasone nonsuppression associated with mood disorders appears to be hypersecretion of corticotropin-releasing factor (CRF) (Gold et al. 1995), the hypothalamic hormone that stimulates the pituitary to release adrenocorticotropic hormone (ACTH), which in turn stimulates the adrenal cortex to release cortisol. Serotonergic input stimulates secretion both of CRF and ACTH and participates in inhibition by corticosteroids of CRF and ACTH. Noradrenergic influences inhibit CRF production but can stimulate release of ACTH (Brown et al. 1994). A functional deficiency of norepinephrine activity and/or an excess of serotonergic transmission could contribute to dexamethasone nonsuppression (Brown et al. 1994; Rush et al. 1997), the former possibility being supported, in many but not all studies, by a significant correlation between plasma cortisol levels after dexamethasone administration and cerebrospinal fluid (CSF) levels of the norepinephrine metabolite 3-methoxy-4-hydroxyphenylglycol (MHPG) in depressed patients (Brown et al. 1994). An entirely different mechanism is suggested by findings of considerable variability in serum dexamethasone levels between patients taking the same dose of the steroid (Devanand et al. 1991). This observation raises the possibility that in some patients, apparent dexamethasone nonsuppression may actually reflect faster metabolism of dexamethasone, with insufficient levels to provide feedback inhibition of CRF and cortisol production.

Although it may create a window into the physiology of arousal in mood disorders, the DST has not proved useful as a diagnostic tool (Carroll 1986). Dexamethasone nonsuppression can be a response to hospitalization, acute illness, dementia, or recent weight loss. Smoking, alcohol use, and medications that accelerate dexamethasone metabolism can make it more difficult to achieve levels of dexamethasone necessary to suppress cortisol secretion and can therefore increase the number of false-positive results in actual clinical practice. Between 50% and 60% of endogenously depressed patients with normal DST results still have a depressive illness, and without a clinical evaluation it is not possible to differentiate false-negative from false-positive results (Carroll 1986). On the other hand, persistent dexamethasone nonsuppression in a patient with remitted major depression may be a marker of increased risk of relapse if treatment is stopped, and very high cortisol levels after dexamethasone administration (>10 μg/dL) may be a marker of psychosis in depressed patients. The DST has a specificity of 87% and a sensitivity of 48% for distinguishing between melancholic and nonmelancholic depression (Rush et al. 1997), but this is not of great practical importance, given that both types of depression are treated similarly.

Thyrotropin-Releasing Hormone Stimulation Test

There are important reasons for interest in thyroid function in mood disorders. Thyroiditis is more common in patients with mood disorders, and hypothyroidism occurs with increased frequency in rapid-cycling bipolar disorder. Thyroid hormones play an important role in the regulation of biological rhythms as well as neurotransmitter and receptor function (Stancer and Persad 1982). Thyroid dysfunction can induce abnormal fluctuations of monoaminergic systems involved in mood regulation; these fluctuations may occur at normal circulating thyroid hormone levels if central nervous system delivery or processing of thyroid hormones is reduced, levels of thyroid-stimulating hormone (TSH) or thyrotropin-releasing hormone (TRH) are altered, or cycling of the thyroid axis is disrupted (Bauer and Whybrow 1986). TRH (protirelin), the hypothalamic hormone that stimulates release of TSH by the pituitary gland, has direct effects on the central nervous system, including modulation of the actions of serotonin (5-HT) and dopamine, independent of stimulation of the thyroid or pituitary gland (Marangell et al. 1997).

A number of studies have noted an association between hypothyroidism and rapid cycling (Bauer 1997). As many as 60%–92% of patients with rapid cycling, but only one-third as many without rapid cycling, have been found to have hypothyroidism that is not severe enough to cause medical morbidity. Lithium itself may cause rapid cycling by inducing hypothyroidism. Although not all studies find a correlation between thyroid function and rapid cycling, negative results have usually not involved measurement of TSH levels or TRH stimulation tests.

The TRH stimulation test, an assay of the activity of the hypothalamic-pituitary-thyroid axis, involves measuring TSH concentration increases several times after intravenous infusion of a standard dose (usually 500 IU) of protirelin. A TRH-induced increase in TSH levels of more than approximately 30 IU/mL is considered hyperactive, signifying reduced feedback inhibition of the pituitary by thyroid hormone, which often indicates hypothyroidism or primary hyperactivity at the level of the pituitary. If TSH levels increase by less than 5 IU/mL after TRH infusion, the TRH stimulation test result is said to be blunted, in which case feedback inhibition of the pituitary by a hyperactive thyroid gland is excessive or primary pituitary failure has occurred.

About one-third of otherwise euthyroid, melancholic depressed patients have been found to have a blunted TRH stimulation test result (Rush et al. 1997). In some studies this finding has been a state variable, reverting to normal with remission of depression, whereas in other studies it has been a trait variable, remaining abnormal after normalization of mood. In most studies, there is at most a modest likelihood that depressed patients with dexamethasone nonsuppression will also have a blunted TRH stimulation test result (Rush et al. 1997). Conversely, in one study, 74% of patients with melancholic major depression or bipolar depression who had a blunted TRH stimulation test result also had dexamethasone nonsuppression (Rush et al. 1997).

A blunted TRH stimulation test result in melancholic depression is not associated with changes in circulating levels of thyroid hormones, and therefore it is unlikely that the test is a marker of true hyperthyroidism. However, delivery of thyroid hormone to feedback systems in the pituitary and hypothalamus may be excessive. It is also possible that TRH receptors in the pituitary are hypoactive. Chronic overstimulation of these receptors by endogenous TRH might lead to their downregulation but would also result in increased thyroid hormone levels, so a primary defect in cellular signaling seems more likely. The input of serotonergic and noradrenergic tracts to the pituitary could permit a functional deficiency of norepinephrine activity or an excess of serotonergic transmission to alter TSH release and contribute to a blunted TRH stimulation test result (Rush et al. 1997).

Abnormal Circadian Rhythms and Sleep

Depressed mood often has a diurnal variation, and episodes may follow a monthly or seasonal pattern of recurrence. Some mood disorders, such as seasonal affective disorder and rapid-cycling bipolar disorder, are defined by their periodicity. Phase advances (i.e., peaking earlier in the day) have been noted in sleep onset, rapid eye movement (REM) sleep, temperature, and hormonal and neurotransmitter rhythms, including those of concentrations of cortisol, 5-HT, dopamine, and norepinephrine.

Abnormal sleep is one of the most common symptoms of depression, and the most frequent cause of sleep disorders in patients evaluated at sleep centers is depression (Buysse et al. 1997). Well-replicated changes in sleep architecture in MDD include decreased sleep continuity, more awakenings, decreased REM sleep latency (i.e., decreased length of time between the onset of sleep to the first REM cycle), increased REM sleep density (increased number of REMs per unit of time during REM sleep), increased length of time in REM sleep, and difficulty entering and remaining in slow-wave sleep (Rush et al. 1997). Some of the decreased REM sleep latency observed in melancholic depression is primary, and some is secondary to reduced slow-wave sleep, which allows REM sleep to shift to the earlier part of the night (Kupfer 1995). Deficiencies in sleep efficiency and slow-wave sleep may explain why depressed patients sometimes feel tired even if they appear to sleep excessively.

Abnormalities of sleep architecture have been most notable in melancholic depression and in bipolar and psychotic depression, the latter being accompanied by sleep-onset REMs, or a REM sleep latency of less than 20 minutes (Dubovsky and Thomas 1992). However, reduced REM sleep latency has not been found in seasonal affective disorder (Hellekson 1989). Polysomnographic sleep measures were initially thought to be trait variables but more recently have been found to persist after clinical remission in some cases (Rush et al. 1997). Results may be contradictory because some findings (such as decreased slow-wave sleep) are trait variables, whereas others (such as decreased sleep continuity, decreased REM sleep latency, and increased phasic REM activity) are state variables.

Any single abnormality of sleep architecture is not strongly associated with major depression (Rush et al. 1997). For example, reduced REM sleep latency has been reported in 20%–40% of nondepressed patients (Thase et al. 1997). On the other hand, the triad of reduced REM sleep latency, increased REM sleep density, and decreased sleep efficiency reliably discriminated between patients with MDD and control subjects in a carefully controlled study (Thase et al. 1997). Even in this study, however, 55% of depressed outpatients had no abnormalities according to any of the three measures, which makes the sleep electroencephalogram a poor diagnostic test.

Attempts have been made to correlate polysomnographic findings with treatment outcome in MDD. Treatment with antidepressants delays REM sleep onset, decreases total REM sleep, and shifts slow-wave sleep earlier in the night (Buysse et al. 1997). When slow-wave sleep occupies a more normal position (that is, occurs earlier in the night), patients feel more rested, whereas a shift of REM sleep to the latter part of the night and closer to the time of awakening can cause patients to remember more of their dreams. When suppression of REM sleep by antidepressants leads to REM rebound, dreams may become disturbingly vivid.

As presumed markers of a "biological" influence, sleep findings such as decreased REM sleep latency have been said to predict a poorer response to psychotherapy, although this impression was not confirmed in controlled studies (Thase et al. 1997). On the other hand, Thase et al. (1997) found that the triad mentioned earlier of reduced REM sleep latency, increased REM sleep density, and decreased sleep efficiency, but not any single measure, predicted a poorer response to interpersonal and cognitive-behavioral psychotherapy for major depression. It has also been reported that failure of slow-wave sleep to increase or at least shift to earlier in the night in response to any kind of treatment predicts a higher risk of relapse or recurrence (Buysse et al. 1997).

Hypotheses about mechanisms of the complex changes in sleep architecture in major depression are incomplete. In cases of early-morning awakening and decreased REM sleep latency, there appears to be a phase advance of the sleep–wake cycle, which is driven by the weak oscillator that also drives activity–rest cycles; and of the REM cycle, which is dependent on the strong oscillator that also controls body temperature. Because muscarinic cholinergic systems increase REM sleep, cholinergic excess could be one cause of increased REM sleep density and increased time in REM sleep (Rush et al. 1997). However, decreased REM sleep latency could also be a function of noradrenergic deficiency. Changes in REM sleep may be secondary to a disturbance of non-REM sleep, which is regulated by corticothalamic circuits (Buysse et al. 1997).

A hypothesis that integrates alterations in circadian rhythms and psychosocial events holds that negative or positive experiences represent changes in social zeitgebers that disrupt social rhythms and destabilize circadian rhythms (Ashman et al. 1999). Studies of major social zeitgebers in mood disorders have found that depression and anxiety are associated with reduced stability of timing of these activities (Ashman et al. 1999). Dysregulation of mood in MDD could be related to a phase advance or at least desynchronization of the strong oscillator with respect to the weak oscillator. Loss of predictability of circadian rhythms—with reduced amplitude of rhythms of body temperature, cortisol, melatonin, and norepinephrine—could suggest impaired entrainment of these rhythms. Antidepressants restore normal organization of circadian rhythms and resynchronize the two oscillators, but it is not clear whether this is a therapeutic mechanism or a marker of overall improvement in psychobiology.

Destabilization of the sleep–wake cycle in particular may be a precipitant of bipolar episodes (Ashman et al. 1999), especially rapid cycling (Wirz-Justice et al. 1999). This possibility was addressed in a study involving 9 patients with rapid-cycling bipolar disorder (Ashman et al. 1999). Seventeen specific social events were recorded each day in order to compute indexes of the number of daily activities, rhythmicity (stability of timing of daily activities), and the time spent socially isolated. Compared with age- and sex-matched control subjects, patients had less rhythmicity of daily activities and lower activity levels. Especially when they were depressed, patients were less likely to eat meals, exercise, start work, watch television, or take a nap, and they were later in getting out of bed, eating breakfast, contacting another person, going outside, and having lunch. The daily routines of patients with rapid cycling, therefore, were less organized than those of control subjects. In another study, in which 11 women with rapid-cycling bipolar disorder kept sleep logs for 18 months, decreased sleep was the best predictor of mania or hypomania, whereas depression was not associated with any predictable change in sleep (Leibenluft 1996).

Clinical Uses of Biological Tests

Laboratory tests are useful for examining the pathophysiology of mood disorders, but the large numbers of false-positive and false-negative results make them relatively ineffective for diagnosing mood disorders. In addition, no laboratory test can outperform the gold-standard clinical interview to which it is referenced, and no studies exist in which diagnosis was prospectively predicted by laboratory test results alone. A single laboratory test such as the DST can occasionally be used to predict the risk of a relapse if an antidepressant is withdrawn or to increase the index of suspicion of psychosis in refractory depression. However, studies of correlations between multiple tests may create a better window into the complex phenomenology of mood disorders.

The DST, the TRH stimulation test, and sleep electroencephalography can distinguish between melancholic and nonmelancholic major depression but not between bipolar and unipolar depression (Rush et al. 1997). For identifying melancholic depression, a blunted TRH stimulation test result has the greatest specificity and the least sensitivity, whereas shortened REM sleep latency has the greatest sensitivity and the least specificity (Rush et al. 1997). The sensitivity and specificity of any of these tests can be adjusted by altering the cutoff point for a positive test result. For example, using a cortisol level (after dexamethasone administration) of 10 μg/dL as a positive result will increase the number of true-positive results as well as the number of false-negative results. However, at least one-fourth of patients with endogenous major depression demonstrate no abnormality on any of the three tests (Rush et al. 1997).

Ultimately, biological tests may prove most useful for identifying specific dimensions of mood disorders that may indicate specific treatments or combinations of them. For example, inhibitors of the hypothalamic-pituitary-adrenal axis might be useful for patients with refractory depression and excessive release of CRF, whereas manipulations of the sleep–wake cycle might be effective for patients with prominent disruptions of the relationship between slow-wave and REM sleep. If depressed patients with anxiety were found to have a different pattern of arousal than nonanxious depressed patients, treatments aimed at arousal mechanisms might be specifically helpful.

■ NEUROTRANSMITTERS

Theories linking disordered chemistry to disordered mood go back to at least the fourth century B.C., when Hippocrates hypothesized that mood depends on a balance among the four bodily humors: blood, phlegm, yellow bile, and black bile, found in the heart, brain, liver, and spleen, respectively. Hippocrates proposed that depression was caused by an excess of black bile in the spleen. Because the spleen occupied a position in the body analogous to the position of Saturn in the heavens, it was believed that those born under the sign of Saturn were prone to depression. These ideas are the basis of references to an attitude of depressive hostility as *spleen* and to morose people as *saturnine.*

The conviction that there must be some inherent biodynamic alteration in mood disorders has continued over the years. Herman Boerhaave, a prominent Leiden physician of the eighteenth century, argued that depression was caused by "nervous and melancholy juice." The psychologist William James was equally certain that changes in mood must be accompanied by some form of "chemical action." In his "Project for a Scientific Psychology," Sigmund Freud (1950[1895]/1966) proposed a complex pathophysiological theory based on a hydraulic model of neuronal functioning, which he later abandoned. Modern technology has made it possible to study the "humors" and "melancholy juice" of the twentieth century—neurotransmitters, receptors, and intracellular messengers.

Biogenic Amines

Biologically active (biogenic) amines such as norepinephrine, 5-HT, dopamine, and acetylcholine are neurotransmitters in brain systems that originate in the brain stem. Because these systems modulate background activity of multiple neuronal circuits, it has been proposed that abnormal function of biogenic amines occurs in mood disorders. The monoamine hypothesis, which was first advanced in 1965, holds that monoamines such as norepinephrine and 5-HT are deficient in depression and that the therapeutic action of antidepressants depends on increasing synaptic availability of these monoamines (Schildkraut 1965). The monoamine hypothesis was based on observations that antidepressants block reuptake inhibition of norepinephrine, 5-HT, and/or dopamine. However, inferring neurotransmitter pathophysiology from an observed action of a class of medications on neurotransmitter availability is similar to concluding that because aspirin causes gastrointestinal bleeding, headaches are caused by too much blood and the therapeutic action of aspirin in headaches is the production of blood loss.

Additional experience has not confirmed the monoamine hypothesis (Salomon et al. 1997). Monoamine precursors such as tyrosine or tryptophan by themselves do not reliably improve mood. Depletion of 5-HT can aggravate depression that has been in remission, but it does not predictably cause depression, and when it does cause depression, the depression is not sustained. Some substances that are monoamine reuptake inhibitors, such as amphetamines and cocaine, do not have reliable antidepressant properties, and antidepressant medications exist (e.g., iprindole, mianserin, mirtazapine, ketanserin) that have no effect on monoamine reuptake. In the case of monoamine reuptake inhibitors that are antidepressants, reuptake inhibition is immediate, whereas the onset of antidepressant effect is delayed a month or more. Tianeptine, a tricyclic antidepressant that enhances 5-HT reuptake and reduces synaptic 5-HT is as effective an antidepressant as the serotonin reuptake inhibitors, which have the opposite effect.

Neurotransmitter reuptake inhibition may not predict antidepressants' therapeutic effects, but it does predict side effects. Norepinephrine is a neurotransmitter in arousal centers such as the locus coeruleus and in the sympathetic nervous system. Medications that increase noradrenergic activity can produce anxiety, tremor, tachycardia, diaphoresis, insomnia, and related symptoms of arousal. Because 5-HT influences gastrointestinal motility, cerebral vasomotor tone, appetitive functions, and arousal, serotonin reuptake inhibitors can produce nausea, diarrhea, headaches, appetite loss, sexual dysfunction, sedation, and jitteriness. Dopamine is a neurotransmitter of activation, movement, reward, and blood vessel tone, and dopamine reuptake inhibitors tend to be activating and may increase blood pressure.

Norepinephrine

Both relative deficiencies and excesses of central noradrenergic activity have been postulated to exist in depression. An early hypothesis was that decreased activity and motivation in depression was related to reduced noradrenergic tone, and hyperactivity in mania was related to noradrenergic excess. However, reports of increased norepinephrine activity in depression have been more frequent than reports of reduced activity. This is consistent with evidence of high levels of arousal such as dexamethasone nonsuppression or phase advance of circadian rhythms, which are present even in behaviorally slowed depressed patients.

Unmedicated depressed patients do not show consistent changes in α_1-adrenergic receptor numbers (Brown et al. 1994). However, downregulation and hyposensitivity of β- and possibly α_2-adrenergic receptors have been reported (Brown et al. 1994). In animal studies, chronic antidepressant treatment decreases the number of α_2- and β-adrenergic receptors and increases the density of α_1-adrenergic receptors (Brown et al. 1994). The first change would increase norepinephrine release, whereas the second would be expected to reduce adrenergic transmission through postsynaptic receptors. However, although a number of antidepressants downregulate β-adrenergic receptors, ECT upregulates these receptors; and mianserin, an antidepressant in use in Europe, does not affect β-adrenergic receptor density at all (Leonard 1994). Reported actions on other adrenergic receptor subtypes may not be relevant to the therapeutic effect of antidepressants (Brown et al. 1994).

Drawing on studies of responsiveness of noradrenergic measures such as plasma MHPG, a norepinephrine metabolite, to mild stresses, Siever and Davis (1985) suggested that depression is associated not with consistently increased or reduced norepinephrine activity but with uneven responsiveness to stresses that activate noradrenergic stress-response systems. Like the heat produced by a furnace that is controlled by a poorly regulated thermostat, baseline noradrenergic activity is excessive, but acute stresses that call for mobilization of the stress response result in inadequate mobilization of additional noradrenergic transmission. The behavioral and affective correlates of this situation would be high levels of baseline anxiety and a sense of spinning one's wheels and an inability to mount an organized response to important challenges.

Serotonin

Neurons using 5-HT, which is phylogenetically the oldest neurotransmitter, originate in raphe (midline) nuclei in the brain stem and project throughout the brain. These connections and interactions make it possible for 5-HT to interact with other biogenic amines and to contribute to the regulation of many core psychobiological functions that are disrupted in mood disorders, including mood, anxiety, arousal, vigilance, irritability, thinking, cognition, appetites, aggression, circadian and seasonal rhythms, nociception, and neuroendocrine functions. 5-HT may serve as a "neurochemical brake" on certain innate behaviors that are normally suppressed, such as aggression, including aggression turned against the self. Therefore, it is not surprising that serotonergic dysfunction has been implicated in mood disorders and that medications that act on 5-HT are useful in the treatment of mood disorders.

5-HT mediates its diverse actions through multiple receptors with different second messenger signaling mechanisms. At least 15 distinct 5-HT receptor subtypes have been identified, many with further functional subtypes (e.g., 5-HT$_{1A}$, 5-HT$_{1D}$) (Dubovsky and Thomas 1995). More is known about some of these receptors than others. For example, 5-HT$_1$ receptors use cyclic adenosine monophosphate (cAMP) and mediate functions such as body temperature, anxiety, and nociception. Subtypes of the 5-HT$_2$ receptor, which signal via the phosphatidylinositol (PI) system (described in "Second Messengers"), mediate psychosis, mood, sleep, vasomotor tone, and platelet aggregation; 5-HT$_2$ heteroreceptors on postsynaptic dopamine D$_2$ receptors influence activity of postsynaptic D$_2$ receptors. The 5-HT$_3$ receptor is linked directly to an ion channel and influences anxiety, psychosis, and nausea; a 5-HT$_3$ heteroreceptor on limbic dopaminergic neurons helps to mediate substance reward. Because the functions of most other receptors, as well as the action of medications on these receptors, have not been well studied in psychiatry, not all the roles they play in mood disorders are known.

A number of studies have found lower concentrations of 5-hydroxyindoleacetic acid (5-HIAA, the major 5-HT metabolite) in the CSF of depressed patients than in the CSF of control subjects (Brown et al. 1994). The finding of reduced platelet 5-HT uptake in unmedicated major depression (Brown et al. 1994) could represent hypofunction of a cellular 5-HT transporter. If a similar malfunction existed in the brain, it could result in reduced 5-HT stores, or reduction of 5-HT uptake could be a means of compensating for increased 5-HT availability. In favor of the former hypothesis, this transporter is downregulated after chronic depletion of 5-HT (Vawter et al. 2000). Decreased binding of [^{3}H]imipramine, a marker of the 5-HT uptake site, has been inconsistently found in platelets of unmedicated depressed patients (Brown et al. 1994). Additionally, no change in platelet binding of [^{3}H]paroxetine, which may be a better marker of the 5-HT uptake site, has been found in major depression (Brown et al. 1994). Many platelet 5-HT findings may be confounded by seasonal and circadian variations in platelet 5-HT uptake (Brown et al. 1994). Reduced [^{3}H]imipramine binding has been found in the brains of depressed patients who committed suicide or died of natural causes, but this finding has been inconsistent (Brown et al. 1994); and another postmortem study found decreased 5-HT uptake sites, as measured by [^{3}H]citalopram, in both major depression and bipolar disorder (Vawter et al. 2000). A more reliable finding has been increased numbers of platelet 5-HT$_2$ receptor sites, consistent with a reduction in systemic serotonergic activity (McBride et al. 1994). Conversely, using the polymerase chain reaction technique, no association was found between polymorphisms of the 5-HT$_{1A}$ and 5-HT$_{2C}$ receptor genes and depression, mania, delusions, or disorganization in patients with unipolar or bipolar mood disorder (Serretti et al. 2000).

A strategy to assess serotonergic function indirectly in mood disorders involves depletion of tryptophan, the amino acid precursor of 5-HT. Some studies have shown that tryptophan-depleting diets produce acute but brief relapses of depression in patients with remitted depression but have no behavioral effect in healthy subjects (Salomon et al. 1997). Another indirect approach uses neuroendocrine probes of the serotonergic system. For example, the

5-HT precursors L-tryptophan and 5-hydroxytryptophan and the serotonin releaser and reuptake inhibitor fenfluramine release hormones under serotonergic control, such as cortisol, growth hormone, and prolactin (Brown et al. 1994). Findings of blunted release of prolactin in response to tryptophan and fenfluramine in some patients with major depression have been interpreted as indicating primary subsensitivity of postsynaptic 5-HT receptors located on prolactin-releasing cells (Brown et al. 1994). However, these kinds of neuroendocrine challenges are not selective for serotonergic systems, and variations in methodology limit generalizability of findings. In addition, whereas studies of prolactin response to serotonergic provocation suggest postsynaptic 5-HT receptor subsensitivity in major depression, cortisol release studies suggest the opposite (Brown et al. 1994).

Reduction of concentrations of central 5-HT and its metabolites may not be a marker of depression so much as a feature that commonly accompanies depression. Of 7 studies, 5 demonstrated modestly reduced brain stem 5-HT and 5-HIAA levels in people, regardless of diagnosis, who committed suicide (Mann et al. 1989). In 10 of 15 studies of CSF 5-HIAA, levels were lower in depressed patients who made a suicide attempt than in those who did not attempt suicide (Mann et al. 1989). Increased binding of labeled markers to 5-HT_2 and 5-HT_{1A} receptors in the frontal cortex of individuals who committed suicide suggests that these receptors were upregulated to compensate for decreased synaptic availability of 5-HT in suicide (Buchsbaum et al. 1997). A study involving 22 drug-free depressed inpatients with a history of a suicide attempt found that current depressive episodes in patients whose past attempts caused more medical damage and were better planned were associated with lower CSF 5-HIAA concentrations (but no changes in levels of other neurotransmitter metabolites) than were depressive episodes in patients who had made less lethal and less well planned suicide attempts, which suggests that reduced 5-HIAA levels may be a marker of seriousness of suicidal ideation (Mann and Malone 1997). In a study involving 237 patients with mood disorders and 187 control subjects, a variant of the 5-HT transporter gene was associated with violent but not other kinds of suicide attempts (Bellivier et al. 2000).

Reduced central serotonergic activity was originally thought to be specific for depression and then for suicidal depression, but this finding appears to be correlated with violent and/or impulsive suicidal behavior, whether the descriptive diagnosis is depression, schizophrenia, behavior disorder, or personality disorder (Mann et al. 1989; McBride et al. 1994). Reduced serotonergic tone is not even restricted to suicidality per se but is also associated with loss of control over many forms of impulsivity and/or aggression, regardless of whether they are directed inward or outward (Mann et al. 1989).

Considered together, studies of 5-HT in major depression suggest both hypofunction and hyperfunction (Brown et al. 1994; Leonard 1994). Findings such as decreased 5-HT and 5-HIAA levels in postmortem brain and CSF studies, brief relapse of depression with diets that deplete 5-HT precursors, decreased postsynaptic 5-HT receptor sensitivity in depression, and the existence of antidepressant properties of some medications that enhance serotonergic transmission suggest underactivity of serotonergic systems. Conversely, decreased platelet 5-HT uptake in depression, increased 5-HT$_2$ receptor binding in the frontal cortex of individuals who have committed suicide, and reduction of postsynaptic 5-HT$_2$ binding and CSF 5-HIAA levels with chronic antidepressant treatment suggest increased serotonergic transmission in major depression.

One reason for this uncertainty is that neurobiological and pharmacological studies generally emphasize isolated aspects of serotonergic function, although in the intact organism the activity of this neurotransmitter cannot be separated from the action of other transmitters. For example, 5-HT is a cotransmitter with γ-aminobutyric acid (GABA) and norepinephrine. Serotonergic and noradrenergic neurons can take up each other's transmitter, altering the functioning of the parent neuron. Raphe serotonergic neurons inhibit noradrenergic neurons in the locus coeruleus and regulate β-adrenergic receptor number and function. Conversely, agonists of α- and β-adrenergic receptors and GABA$_B$ receptors alter the function of several 5-HT receptors.

Many other 5-HT interactions have been identified. Raphe serotonergic neurons synapse with nigrostriatal and mesolimbic dopaminergic neurons, and dopaminergic neurons have 5-HT receptors that permit tonic control of dopamine release in the midbrain, striatum, and nucleus accumbens. Depending on the circumstances, 5-HT may facilitate dopamine release in the nucleus accumbens (via 5-HT$_3$ heteroreceptors) and inhibit dopaminergic activity in the striatum (via 5-HT$_2$ heteroreceptors). Serotonergic neurons have glucocorticoid receptors that alter gene transcription, perhaps providing a feedback loop that permits serotonergic systems to modulate the stress response (Leonard 1994).

In evaluating the effect of new serotonergic medications, it is important to bear in mind that medications such as selective serotonin reuptake inhibitors are not so much specific treatments for MDD as therapies for any syndrome that involves dysregulated mood, anxiety, impulsive and self-destructive behavior, circadian rhythm disturbance, or appetitive dysfunction. Similarly, drugs that antagonize the 5-HT$_2$ receptor, such as clozapine, may have applications in a variety of disorders characterized by dysregulated thought and mood. Until validated rating scales for serotonergic functions are used along with instruments for categorical diagnosis (e.g., Structured Clinical Interview for DSM-IV or SCID-IV) in treatment outcome studies, the precise spectrum of action of serotonergic medications will not be fully explored.

Dopamine

Some investigations have found that CSF concentrations of the dopamine metabolite homovanillic acid are lower in patients with major depression than in control subjects and that lower CSF homovanillic acid levels are found in more severely depressed patients, but results have not been consistent (Brown et al. 1994). The dopamine reuptake inhibitors nomifensine (no longer available), amineptine (available in Europe), and bupropion are antidepressants. Dopaminergic agonists such as bromocriptine, pramipexole, and piribedil, as well as the dopamine-releasing stimulants methylphenidate and dextroamphetamine, have antidepressant properties that make them useful adjuncts in the treatment of depression (Brown et al. 1994).

As is true of 5-HT, any apparent dopaminergic hypofunction may have a greater effect on dimensions of mood disorders than on specific diagnoses. Because mobilization of goal-directed behavior is mediated by dopamine, underactivity of dopaminergic systems may be related to decreased drive and motivation in depression (Brown et al. 1994). Underresponsive dopaminergic systems could be one reason for anhedonia in depressed patients. Given that increased levels of dopamine metabolites have been observed in psychotic depression, hyperactivity of dopaminergic motivational and action systems could be related to manic or psychotic symptoms in mood disorders.

Substance P

Speculations have arisen that substance P could mediate the psychological pain of depression as well as physical pain. Substance P is a neuropeptide involved in the mediation of nociception and more generically in awareness of the intensity of aversive stimuli. A role of substance P in depression is suggested by findings that substance P is also involved in CNS pathways for psychological stress and possibly for anxiety and depression and reports of different distributions of neurkin 1 (NK1) substance P receptors subtypes in the anterior cingulate cortex of patients with depression compared with control subjects and with patients with other disorders. Such findings have led to trials of NK1 antagonists in major depressive disorder described in the "Novel Treatments" section of Chapter 4.

γ-Aminobutyric Acid

GABA is the major inhibitory neurotransmitter in the central nervous system. Inadequate GABAergic input to noradrenergic arousal systems could lead to the kind of unrestrained arousal that characterizes mood disorders. Decreased CSF GABA levels have been reported in major depression (Leonard 1994), and some antidepressants increase the number of GABA$_B$ receptor sites in rat brain (Leonard 1994). Benzodiazepines, which increase the affinity of GABA$_B$ receptors for endogenous GABA, are usually thought to aggravate depression, but this class of medications can reduce depressive symptoms in patients who are anxious and depressed. Gabapentin, an anticonvulsant with unclear GABAergic actions, has both anxiolytic and antidepressant actions, although reduction of depression could be secondary to decreased anxiety in these situations. Because GABA$_B$ receptors may act as heteroreceptors on serotonergic terminals in limbic regions (Leonard 1994) in addition to moderating noradrenergic output, any pathophysiological contribution of GABA and any therapeutic effect of GABAergic medications in mood disorders may ultimately be mediated by other neurotransmitter systems.

Acetylcholine

It has been hypothesized that cholinergic transmission, relative to noradrenergic transmission, is excessive in depression and inadequate in mania. Because acetylcholine is a neurotransmitter in structures that mediate withdrawal and punishment such as the periventricular system, cholinergic hyperactivity could increase withdrawal behavior in depression. In support of this hypothesis are the findings that cholinergic input reduces REM sleep latency (decreased REM sleep latency is seen in depression), some antidepressants have anticholinergic properties, lecithin (an acetylcholine precursor) and cholinesterase inhibitors such as physostigmine and donepezil reduce mania in some patients and sometimes replace mania with depression, and cholinergic rebound after abrupt withdrawal of anticholinergic medications can cause relapse of depression (Dilsaver and Coffman 1989). The observation that patients with bipolar disorder smoke as frequently as patients with schizophrenia could be interpreted as indicating an antimanic action of nicotinic receptor stimulation, but if smoking is a form of self-treatment for bipolar disorder, it could correct dysfunction of information processing. Lithium was thought to induce upregulation of cholinergic receptors, but this finding has been contested (Lerer and Stanley 1985). In contrast to earlier suggestions of the existence of muscarinic receptor supersensitivity in depression, no change in muscarinic receptor number was found in the brains of people who committed suicide (Kaufmann et al. 1984). Additional objections raised against the cholinergic hypothesis include observations that not all anticholinergic medications are antidepressants, none of the newer antidepressants is anticholinergic, and muscarinic receptors were initially considered in testing the hypothesis, although most agents used to test the hypothesis act on nicotinic receptors.

Interactions of Neurotransmitter Systems

Early attempts to understand the role of neurotransmitters and their receptors involved the hypothesis that some depressions were characterized by functional norepinephrine deficiency, whereas others were associated with serotonergic hypofunction. According to this hypothesis, low norepinephrine depression would respond preferentially to noradrenergic antidepressants, and low 5-HT depressions would respond better to treatments that enhance availability of that neurotransmitter. This prediction was never confirmed, and no evidence of differing "serotonergic" and "noradrenergic" depressive subtypes has emerged (Brown et al. 1994). The hypothesis was then revised (and termed the *permissive amine hypothesis*) to include the concept that serotonergic deficiency contributes to most cases of depression, some of which have additional noradrenergic dysfunction (Vawter et al. 2000). This hypothesis predicted that antidepressants improve coordination between neurotransmitter systems.

These kinds of speculations underscore the overlap of dimensional features of depression perhaps linked to interactions among neurotransmitter systems. When arousal associated with noradrenergic excess is sufficient to overwhelm regulation of aggression and impulsivity that has been impaired by suboptimally active serotonergic systems, the predominant problem may be suicide, various forms of outwardly directed aggression, or generalized impulsivity, whether the primary diagnosis is a mood disorder, an anxiety disorder, schizophrenia, or a personality disorder. Inadequate function of serotonergic systems that regulate intrusive thought may interact with disturbances of mood to produce ruminative depressive states or racing thoughts that remain stuck on a particular idea. If the interaction is with the consequences of traumatic experiences, the intrusive recall of posttraumatic stress disorder may develop if serotonergic systems that regulate recurrent thoughts and arousal do not function normally. Dysregulation of thought processes is a feature of schizophrenia, and when this dysregulation interacts with the psychobiology of mood, the same malfunction may figure in psychotic depression, bipolar illness, and schizoaffective disorder.

In addition to being derived from research that ignores neurotransmitter interactions and evidence of dysregulation of multiple systems in mood disorders, traditional neurotransmitter hypotheses are difficult to apply to bipolar mood disorders. For example, if mania is associated primarily with neurotransmitter changes (e.g., increased norepinephrine and dopaminergic activity) that are the opposites of changes in depression, why are almost 50% of manic patients depressed at the same time that they are manic (i.e., why do they have mixed mania)? And how could neurotransmitter activity change direction so abruptly and rapidly if such activity were driving ultradian (ultrarapid) cycling?

These contradictions are more readily understood if one appreciates that all neurotransmitters and receptors that have been studied in mood disorders interact with and influence each other (Brown et al. 1994; Leonard 1994). Cotransmission using more than one neurotransmitter in the same neuron is the rule. Most cerebral functions are the result of the converging action of many different neurotransmitters. For example, excitability in the human cortex is regulated by acetylcholine, GABA, norepinephrine, histamine, and purines, in addition to 5-HT. Each of these transmitters may produce more than one postsynaptic signal in the same neuron by activating interacting receptors, and more than one transmitter may induce the same change in postsynaptic neurons. This kind of overlap provides a mechanism for fine-tuning complex adaptations to multiple kinds of input.

Such interactions make it unlikely that the pathophysiology of mood disorders can be linked to any single neurotransmitter. Instead, different aspects of the psychobiological malfunctions in mood disorders may be related to different kinds of neurotransmitter dysfunctions (Brown et al. 1994; Leonard 1994). For example, disordered noradrenergic function may be related to anxiety, agitation, and excessive arousal, whereas loss of dopaminergic function could lead to deficits in mobilizing goal-directed behaviors and emotional incentives. Loss of serotonergic regulation of aggression would be best correlated with anxiety, rumination, appetitive dysfunction, and violent, dangerous, and/or impulsive suicidal behavior; and excessive cholinergic tone could lead to withdrawal and experiencing of events as punitive. It is likely that other neurotransmitters and neuromodulators such as neuropeptides and prostaglandins are also dysregulated, contributing to increased intensity of dysphoric affect.

Rather than being related to any particular neurotransmitter disturbance, then, mood disorders may be disorders of the overall cohesiveness of multiple transmitter systems involved in responding to danger. Antidepressant therapies do not affect one of these systems but produce adaptational changes in multiple neurotransmitter systems (Leonard 1994). Greater coordination among affective, cognitive, and behavioral systems associated with these transmitters may be associated with normalization of mental state.

Second Messengers

Simultaneous loss of regulation of multiple neurotransmitter systems, or multiple downstream effects of loss of regulation of a single neurotransmitter system, do not on the surface explain the complex pathophysiology of mood disorders, especially if one must postulate opposing neurotransmitter changes at the same time in patients with mixed bipolar syndromes. Given that there are many neurotransmitters and neuromodulators and many more receptors, an alternative hypothesis is that one or more of the few second messengers that mediate diverse neurotransmitter and receptor actions are poorly regulated. The bidirectional actions of second messengers allow unitary changes in second messenger function to produce diverse changes in transmitter synthesis and release and in receptor activity, leading to complex neurotransmitter and receptor effects. At a cellular level, destabilization of synaptic regulatory mechanisms may be mediated by the loss of the capacity of second messenger systems to maintain cellular signaling within a range that controls oscillations of mood-regulating systems and systems with which they interact.

Three primary second messenger families have been well studied. cAMP acts as an intracellular messenger by activating protein kinase A, which phosphorylates proteins. The PI system is a self-recycling cascade of membrane phospholipids in which phosphatidylinositol 4,5-bisphosphate is hydrolyzed to inositol 1,4,5-triphosphate (IP_3) and diacylglycerol by phospholipase C. IP_3 releases calcium ions (Ca^{2+}) from intracellular stores and contributes to influx of Ca^{2+} from the extracellular space, whereas diacylglycerol activates a ubiquitous intracellular enzyme called protein kinase C. In the presence of Ca^{2+}, protein kinase C phosphorylates many enzymes involved in processes implicated in mood disorders. In addition, entry of positively charged calcium ions produces the plateau phase of the action potential and determines the duration of neuronal action. Different receptors may use different second messengers. For example, the α_1-adrenergic receptor primarily uses cAMP signaling, and the dopamine D_2 receptor and 5-HT_2 receptor increase PI turnover, resulting in an increase in free intracellular Ca^{2+} concentration ($[Ca^{2+}]_i$). The 5-HT_3 and $GABA_A$ receptors are linked directly to ion channels that alter neuronal excitability.

Many second messenger effector systems are linked to their receptors through a guanyl-nucleotide-binding protein (G protein). Receptor occupation leads to hydrolysis of the G protein, which in turn produces the sequence of events that mobilizes second messengers. A single receptor may be associated with more than one G protein, permitting a neurotransmitter to activate more than one second messenger. The same G protein may be associated with more than one receptor, enabling the G protein to integrate signals from different transmitters.

Because of the biphasic action of the intracellular calcium ion and its role in kindling, the PI/Ca^{2+} second messenger system has been of interest to investigators studying bipolar mood disorders. $[Ca^{2+}]_i$ is normally regulated very tightly at around 100 nM, or 1/10,000 the Ca^{2+} concentration in the extracellular fluid. Modest increases in $[Ca^{2+}]_i$ accelerate many intracellular actions, whereas greater increases can inhibit the same actions. In addition, the same $[Ca^{2+}]_i$ increase can inhibit a function in one system and activate another function in some other location. Excessive signaling by this messenger, inhibiting some neuronal processes and activating others at the same time, could explain two aspects of bipolar mood disorders that have been difficult to understand—namely, mixtures of manic and depressive symptoms in the same patient and rapid alternations between mania and depression in rapid-cycling bipolar disorder.

In a number of studies, resting and agonist (including 5-HT)-stimulated $[Ca^{2+}]_i$ was increased in platelets and lymphocytes of affectively ill manic patients and depressed bipolar disorder patients but not in platelets of depressed patients with unipolar disorder, control subjects, or bipolar disorder patients who were euthymic after treatment with various medications or ECT (Dubovsky et al. 1992; Okamoto et al. 1995). In vitro incubation with lithium (Dubovsky et al. 1991) or carbamazepine (Dubovsky et al. 1994) decreases platelet $[Ca^{2+}]_i$ significantly in ill patients with bipolar disorder but not in control subjects or euthymic bipolar disorder patients. Carbamazepine, lithium, and lamotrigine have calcium antagonist properties, and lithium reduces hyperactive PI turnover, in part by inhibiting a key but not rate-limiting enzyme called inositol-1-monophosphatase (Dubovsky et al. 1992). As discussed in Chapters 4 and 7, calcium-channel blockers such as verapamil and nimodipine have antimanic properties.

Excessive intracellular calcium signaling could be caused by increased mobilization of stored intracellular Ca^{2+} (which could result from increased IP_3 production) and/or by increased influx of calcium ions. Any of these processes could be caused by increased G protein activity. Hyperactivity of G proteins and of G protein–linked phospholipase C has been found in mononuclear leukocytes and platelets of patients with bipolar disorder and in postmortem brain samples from patients with bipolar disorder who died of various causes (Mathews et al. 1997). The additional observations that β-adrenergic, muscarinic, and dopamine receptor–coupled G protein activity is reversibly increased in mania (Schreiber and Avissar 2000), cortical G protein activity is increased in brains of patients with bipolar disorder (Vawter et al. 2000), and lithium blunts the G protein response to stimulation in animal studies (Avissar and Schreiber 1992) suggest that increased Ca^{2+} signaling may be the effector arm of a cascade of intracellular events that begins with G protein hyperactivity and that is corrected with antimanic drugs. Antidepressants affect G proteins and other aspects of the second messenger cascade (Leonard 1994), and ECT was found to normalize reduced stimulatory and inhibitory G protein activity in mononuclear leukocytes of patients with unipolar depression (Avissar et al. 1998). Signaling systems such as the PI/Ca^{2+} system that are activated by dysregulated mood may contribute to abnormal expression—reported of genes such as the c-*fos* tumor promoter gene and genes for nerve growth factor 1A, glucocorticoid receptors, brain-derived neurotrophic factor, preproenkephalin, and N-methyl-D-aspartate receptor subunits, among others—the net effect of which is to reduce expression of neuroprotective proteins and increase expression of proteins that disrupt regulation of cellular function.

Other Changes in Intracellular Functioning and Medication Effects

A growing understanding of the importance of intracellular mechanisms is stimulating research into additional basic actions of the neuron. One finding is that cell adhesion molecules and synaptic regulatory proteins are altered in both bipolar disorder and MDD (Vawter et al. 2000). Antidepressants in various classes upregulate expression of messenger RNA of the neuroprotective enzyme superoxide dismutase, indicating that these medications can regulate genetic expression (Li et al. 2000). Animal studies and human neuronal tissue studies suggest that antimanic drugs as diverse in structure as valproate and lithium inhibit protein kinase C in addition to altering genetic expression (Manji et al. 1999). The latter actions of lithium and valproate include increased expression of the cytoprotective protein bcl-2 and of the AP-1 family of transcription factors and of a reporter gene driven by an AP-1 promotor, resulting in increases in expression of proteins regulated by these genes (Manji et al. 1999).

■ PSYCHOLOGICAL FACTORS

As is true of biological data, there is less disagreement about whether specific psychological dimensions of mood disorders exist than about whether they are etiological. Proving that a particular psychological factor is causal would require prospectively following people at risk for depression to see whether those with the factor are more likely to develop a mood disorder. A finding that patients who have already had an affective episode and who exhibit the factor in question are more likely to have a recurrence could simply imply that the factor is a residual symptom of the index episode and not an independent risk factor. Even if expensive and difficult prospective studies of psychological risk factors identified a trait that predicted the later onset of depression, the psychological factor might be a marker of a change in biology.

Because none of the psychological theories of mania (e.g., that it is a defense against depression) has ever been tested empirically, we will focus on psychological hypotheses regarding depression.

Abnormal Reactions to Loss

Loss is the life event that has been most reliably linked to depression. Sigmund Freud (1917[1915]/1957) pointed out that both grief and depression are reactions to loss but that depressive symptoms include guilt and low self-esteem. Based on psychoanalytic experience with depressed patients, Freud believed that grieving turned into depression when the bereaved felt ambivalent about the lost object (i.e., person) and could not tolerate the negative side of the ambivalence. An unconscious attack against an internalized image of the lost object that undermines self-esteem, which depends in part on identification with the lost person, is manifested as depression. Freud thought that early, unresolved losses made the patient more likely to have difficulty dealing with losses as an adult. Later theorists pointed out that loss of anything that represents a person and that is overvalued or ambivalently viewed—a group, a profession, a cherished belief, or an ideal, for example—can result in depression.

In a majority of studies comparing depressed patients with healthy control subjects, childhood loss—especially loss of a parent—has had a positive association with adult depression; in addition, depression is more likely to have its onset after a loss, separation, or disappointment (Bemporad 1988). In primate studies, separation from the mother or from a peer, in the case of animals raised with peers, reliably results in behavioral depression and in the physiology of human depression; separation depression can be prevented or reversed with the use of antidepressants. Separation during infancy from the mother or from the peer group also notably increases the risk of adult separation depression (McKinney 1988). Similarly, experience with human infants has demonstrated that early separation can produce a depressive syndrome that predisposes to later depression (Bowlby 1980). Taken together, these kinds of findings suggest a role for loss in the etiology of depression, but the role may involve the physiology as much as the psychology of loss. In particular, disruption of an attachment bond in any primate leads first to distress, which, from an evolutionary standpoint, helps to attract back the parent from whom an infant has been separated. If reunion does not occur promptly, separation distress is replaced by withdrawal, which conserves energy and reduces the chance of attack by a predator. Early separations may sensitize arousal and withdrawal systems to react excessively to subsequent losses, whether real or symbolic.

Although the association between depression and loss seems reliable, it is not as strong as was originally thought. Not only does loss account for only a relatively small portion of the variance in the risk of depression, but also losses of one kind or another precede many other medical and psychiatric illnesses. Loss, an event that is stressful in itself and that removes an important external source of regulation of disrupted psychology and physiology, may be a more severe instance of a range of stresses that predispose to mood disorders.

Other Psychodynamic Theories

Psychoanalyst Karl Abraham postulated that depression is a manifestation of aggression turned against the self in a patient who is unable to express anger against loved ones. Attacks on the introjected other, who psychologically has become a part of the self, undermine adaptive capacities and produce negative affect. In support of this hypothesis is the fact that many depressed patients have difficulty expressing anger openly, either because they lack self-confidence or because they are afraid of being abandoned by a loved one on whom they are excessively dependent. However, it seems unlikely that anger is converted directly into depression in such individuals, because many depressed patients are openly irritable. A more likely explanation is that dependency, sensitivity to loss, and lack of assertiveness lead depressed people to conceal anger, or even differences of opinion with others, until this anger becomes overwhelming, at which point it intrudes into everyday interactions. This problem may be compounded by intensification of all emotional experience in depression.

A hypothesis (Dubovsky 1997) first clearly articulated by Edward Bibring is that the central psychological fault in depression is loss of self-esteem. According to this hypothesis, the depression-prone person is an overambitious, conventional individual with unrealistically high ego ideals. Depression represents deflation of self-confidence and vitality within the self that results from failing to live up to internalized standards that are essential to the patient's self-concept. This concept was expanded in self theory, which emphasizes the central role of the self as an organizer and driving force of all mental functions. Without coherence, mental activities are fragmented and ineffective. Without a sense of vitality, there is inadequate psychic fuel for optimism and useful engagement with challenges and stress. In this formulation, depression is organized around a sense of depletion of the self.

It is traditionally held that the premorbid personality of the depressed patient is perfectionistic, involving high expectations of the self and others. However, this opinion is based primarily on retrospective recall by patients, which is likely to be influenced by their current mental states. Low self-esteem is a symptom of depression, but it has not yet been demonstrated to be a cause. On the other hand, unrealistic expectations and perceptions of the self and others are also invoked in cognitive theories of depression, which employ more objective measures and more formal studies of such expectations and perceptions.

Interpersonal Theory

Four basic interpersonal issues are emphasized in interpersonal theory: unresolved grief, disputes between partners and family members about roles and responsibilities in relationships, transitions to new roles such as the role of a parent or a retired person, and deficits in the social skills that are necessary to sustain a relationship (Klerman et al. 1984). As in other psychodynamic theories, depressed mood and altered biology are hypothesized to be responses to loss or the threat of loss. A psychotherapy derived from interpersonal theory (i.e., interpersonal therapy [described in Chapter 5]) has been found to be effective as a primary treatment for depression and as an adjunct in the treatment of bipolar disorder, although this does not prove that the etiological concept behind the psychotherapy is accurate.

Cognitive Theory

Cognitive theory, which is related to hypotheses derived from an earlier construct called *rational emotive therapy,* holds that negative thinking is a cause rather than a result of depression (Beck et al. 1985). According to the cognitive model, early experience leads to the development of global negative assumptions called *schemata*. Depressive schemata involve all-or-nothing assumptions such as

- If I'm not completely happy, I'll be totally miserable.
- If something isn't done exactly right, it's worthless.
- If I'm not perfect, I'm a failure.
- If everyone doesn't love me unconditionally, no one loves me at all.
- If I'm not in complete control, I'm helpless.
- If I depend on anyone for anything, I'm totally needy.

As long as experience seems to support a schema—for example, if everything a person does seems to work out, or if a person never leans on anyone else—mood remains unambivalently positive. However, if something happens to contradict an all-or-nothing assumption, it proves globally disruptive to self-confidence, and the negative side of the patient's thinking predominates. Failure in one endeavor makes the patient feel like a complete failure. Becoming ill or otherwise requiring assistance leads the patient to think, "I'm totally needy" or "I can't do anything for myself." These negative beliefs, or negative cognitions, are supported by self-fulfilling prophecies that reinforce negative thinking. For instance, the patient who feels helpless as a result of not having been able to influence the outcome of a complex and difficult situation stops trying to do anything to deal with later, simpler, stresses. When this lack of effort results in subsequent failures, the patient's belief that nothing can be done to influence the environment seems to have been proven. Systematic errors in thinking lead to catastrophic thinking and translation of single negative events to global negative expectations of the self, the environment, and the future (the cognitive triad).

Much of the evidence in favor of the cognitive theory of depression comes from demonstrations that psychotherapy based on the theory (i.e., cognitive therapy [discussed in Chapter 5]) is an effective treatment for major depression. However, cognitive therapy is effective even when patients do not express negative cognitions, and any psychotherapy or antidepressant can reverse depression whether or not negative thinking is formally addressed. In addition, all-or-nothing thinking is characteristic of a number of conditions (e.g., personality disorders) in addition to depression.

Learned Helplessness

A concept related to cognitive theory is *learned helplessness,* which was first clearly demonstrated experimentally by psychologist Martin Seligman (1975). The classic learned helplessness paradigm involves exposing an animal to an inescapable noxious but harmless stimulus such as a mild electrical shock. At first, the animal attempts to flee from the shock, but when escape proves impossible, it lies down and accepts the shock passively. If the situation is changed so that the animal can escape the stimulus (for example, if the investigator removes a barrier that was preventing the animal from leaving the portion of the cage where the shock is applied), the animal continues to act as though it cannot get away. The animal cannot be coaxed away from the shock; only forcibly dragging the animal to safety reverses the learned helplessness behavior. A second instance of learned helplessness develops more readily than a first episode. Learned helplessness that develops in one situation may occur in other situations.

Learned helplessness resembles the passive, withdrawn behavior of depression, and resistance to reversing a negative experience is reminiscent of the self-fulfilling negative expectations of depression. Learned helplessness can be demonstrated in humans (for example, by exposing healthy subjects to an inescapable noxious sound), and subjects who score higher on depression rating scales develop learned helplessness more readily than do those without depressive symptoms (Abramson et al. 1978). In animals, pretreatment with an antidepressant prevents learned helplessness. Considering all these data, it has been postulated that previous experiences with uncontrollable situations create a predisposition to learned helplessness. In response to a new uncontrollable circumstance, more severe learned helplessness develops more rapidly than in the past, resulting in the behaviors and cognitions of depression. Given that learned helplessness is similar to loss in that it involves mixtures of arousal and passivity, it could be built on a similar physiological substrate.

Experimental evidence in favor of the learned helplessness theory of depression may not be that strong. It is not clear that learned helplessness in animals is equivalent to human depression. Human subjects with increased depression scores have not had actual depressive disorders and have not sought treatment for any reason. In addition, depression involves symptoms beyond those of learned helplessness.

Behavioral Theories

Behavioral theories of depression, which are related to learned helplessness, hold that depression is caused by loss of reinforcement of nondepressive behaviors, resulting in deficits in adaptive social behaviors such as assertiveness, responding positively to challenge, and otherwise seeking important reinforcers such as affection, caretaking, and attention (Whybrow et al. 1984). At the same time that environmental rewards are no longer forthcoming with positive behavior (noncontingent reinforcement), the patient's helplessness, expressions of distress, physical complaints, and other depressive behaviors may be rewarded, especially if significant others pay more attention to disability than to competence. Loss removes a major social reinforcer, in addition to rupturing an important attachment bond, and results in depressive behaviors if the patient has not developed an adequate repertoire of adaptive behaviors and does not have other sources of reinforcement. Like negative cognitions, depressive behaviors would be expected to drive a depressed mood.

There is little question that interpersonal rewards influence behavior. If important people pay more attention to expressions of helplessness and inadequacy than to expressions of competence, it may be more rewarding to be depressed than to be healthy. However, it remains to be demonstrated that behavioral factors by themselves can induce depression or that treatment of clinically important depression by behavioral techniques alone is effective.

■ REFERENCES

Abramson LY, Seligman MEP, Teasdale JD: Learned helplessness in humans: critique and reformulation. J Abnorm Psychol 87:49–74, 1978

Ashman SB, Mont TH, Kupfer DJ, et al: Relationship between social rhythms and mood in patients with rapid cycling bipolar disorder. Psychiatry Res 86:1–8, 1999

Avissar S, Schreiber G: Interaction of antibipolar and antidepressant treatments with receptor-coupled G proteins. Pharmacopsychiatry 25:44–50, 1992

Avissar S, Nechamkin Y, Roitman G, et al: Dynamics of ECT normalization of low G protein function and immunoreactivity in mononuclear leukocytes of patients with major depression. Am J Psychiatry 155:666–671, 1998

Bauer MS, Whybrow PC: The effect of changing thyroid function on cyclic affective illness in a human subject. Am J Psychiatry 143:633–636, 1986

Beck AT, Jallon SD, Young JE: Treatment of depression with cognitive therapy and amitriptyline. Arch Gen Psychiatry 42:142–148, 1985

Bellivier F, Szoke A, Henry C, et al: Possible association between serotonin transporter gene polymorphism and violent suicidal behavior in mood disorders. Biol Psychiatry 48:319–322, 2000

Bemporad JR: Psychodynamic models of depression and mania, in Depression and Mania. Edited by Georgotas A, Cancro R. New York, Elsevier, 1988, pp 167–180

Berrettini WH, Ferraro TN, Goldin LR, et al: A linkage study of bipolar illness. Arch Gen Psychiatry 54:27–35, 1997

Bonne O, Krausz Y, Gorfine M, et al: Cerebral hypoperfusion in medication resistant, depressed patients assessed by Tc99m HMPAO SPECT. J Affect Disord 41:163–171, 1996

Bowlby J: Loss: Sadness and Depression. New York, Basic Books, 1980

Brown S-L, Steinberg RL, van Praag HM: The pathogenesis of depression: reconsideration of neurotransmitter data, in Handbook of Depression and Anxiety. Edited by den Boer JA, Sitsen JMA. New York, Marcel Dekker, 1994, pp 317–347

Bruder GE, Fong R, Tenke CE, et al: Regional brain asymmetries in major depression with or without an anxiety disorder: a quantitative electroencephalographic study. Biol Psychiatry 41:939–948, 1997

Buchsbaum MS, Wu J, Siegel BV, et al: Effect of sertraline on regional metabolic rate in patients with affective disorder. Biol Psychiatry 41:15–22, 1997

Buysse DJ, Frank EF, Lowe KK, et al: Electroencephalographic sleep correlates of episode and vulnerability to recurrence in depression. Biol Psychiatry 41:406–418, 1997

Carroll BJ: Informed use of the dexamethasone suppression test. J Clin Psychiatry 47:10–12, 1986

Davidson RJ: Anterior cerebral asymmetry and the nature of emotion. Brain Cogn 20:125–151, 1992

Devanand DP, Sackeim HA, Lo E-S, et al: Serial dexamethasone suppression tests and plasma dexamethasone levels. Arch Gen Psychiatry 48:525–533, 1991

Dilsaver SC, Coffman JA: Cholinergic hypothesis of depression: a reappraisal. J Clin Psychopharmacol 9:173–179, 1989

Doris A, Ebmeier KP, Shajahan P: Depressive illness. Lancet 354:1369–1375, 1999

Dubovsky SL: Mind-Body Deceptions. New York, WW Norton, 1997

Dubovsky SL, Thomas M: Psychotic depression: advances in conceptualization and treatment. Hospital and Community Psychiatry 43:1189–1198, 1992

Dubovsky SL, Thomas M: Beyond specificity: effects of serotonin and serotonergic treatments on psychobiological dysfunction. J Psychosom Res 39:429–444, 1995

Dubovsky SL, Lee C, Christiano J: Lithium decreases platelet intracellular calcium ion concentrations in bipolar patients. Lithium 2:167–174, 1991

Dubovsky SL, Murphy J, Christiano J, et al: The calcium second messenger system in bipolar disorders: data supporting new research directions. J Neuropsychiatry Clin Neurosci 4:3–14, 1992

Dubovsky SL, Thomas M, Hijazi A, et al: Intracellular calcium signalling in peripheral cells of patients with bipolar affective disorder. Eur Arch Psychiatry Clin Neurosci 243:229–234, 1994

Dupont RM, Jernigan TL, Heindel W, et al: Magnetic resonance imaging and mood disorders: localization of white matter and other subcortical abnormalities. Arch Gen Psychiatry 52:747–755, 1995

Egeland JA, Gerhard DS, Pauls D, et al: Bipolar affective disorders linked to DNA markers on chromosome 11. Nature 325:783–787, 1987

Freud S: Mourning and melancholia (1917[1915]), in The Standard Edition of the Complete Psychological Works of Sigmund Freud, Vol 14. Translated and edited by Strachey J. London, Hogarth Press, 1957, pp 237–260

Freud S: Project for a scientific psychology (1950[1895]), in The Standard Edition of the Complete Psychological Works of Sigmund Freud, Vol 1. Translated and edited by Strachey J. London, Hogarth Press, 1966, pp 281–397

Geller B, Todd RD, Luby J, et al: Treatment-resistant depression in children and adolescents. Psychiatr Clin North Am 19:253–265, 1996

Gershon ES: Genetics, in Manic-Depressive Illness. Edited by Goodwin FK, Jamison KR. New York, Oxford University Press, 1990, pp 373–401

Gershon ES, Hamovit J, Guroff I, et al: A family study of schizoaffective, bipolar I, bipolar II, unipolar and normal control probands. Arch Gen Psychiatry 39:1157–1167, 1982

Gold PW, Licinio J, Wong ML, et al: Corticotropin releasing hormone in the pathophysiology of melancholic and atypical depression and the mechanisms of action of antidepressant drugs. Ann N Y Acad Sci 77:716–729, 1995

Gorman JM, Coplan JD: Comorbidity of depression and panic disorder. J Clin Psychiatry 57 (suppl 10):34–41, 1996

Gyulai L, Alavi A, Broich K, et al: I-123 iofetamine single-photon computed emission tomography in rapid cycling bipolar disorder: a clinical study. Biol Psychiatry 41:152–161, 1997

Hellekson C: Phenomenology of seasonal affective disorder: an Alaskan perspective, in Seasonal Affective Disorders and Phototherapy. Edited by Rosenthal NE, Blehar MC. New York, Guilford, 1989, pp 33–43

Jamison KR: Manic-depressive illness, genes, and creativity, in Genetics and Mental Illness: Evolving Issues for Research and Society. Edited by Hall LL. New York, Plenum, 1996, pp 111–132

Joffe RT, Horvath Z, Tarvydas I: Bipolar affective disorder and thalassemia minor (letter). Am J Psychiatry 143:933, 1986

Kaufmann CA, Gillin JC, Hill B, et al: Muscarinic binding in suicides. Psychiatry Res 12:47–55, 1984

Kelsoe JR, Ginns EI, Egeland JA, et al: Re-evaluation of the linkage relationship between chromosome 11p loci and the gene for bipolar affective disorder in the Old Order Amish. Nature 342:238–243, 1989

Kendler KK, Neale MC, Kessler RC, et al: Major depression and generalized anxiety disorder: same genes, (partly) different environments? Arch Gen Psychiatry 49:716–722, 1992

Kendler KK, Kessler CC, Neale MC, et al: The prediction of major depression in women: toward an integrated etiologic model. Am J Psychiatry 150:1139–1148, 1993

Klerman GL, Weissman MM, Rounsaville BJ, et al: Interpersonal Psychotherapy of Depression. New York, Basic Books, 1984

Kupfer DJ: Sleep research in depressive illness: clinical implications—a tasting menu. Biol Psychiatry 38:391–403, 1995

Lavori P, Keller MB, Roth SL: Affective disorders and ABO blood groups: new data and a reanalysis of the literature using the logistic transformation of proportions. J Psychiatr Res 18:119–129, 1984

Leibenluft E: Women with bipolar illness: clinical and research issues. Am J Psychiatry 153:163–173, 1996

Leonard BE: Effect of antidepressants on specific neurotransmitters: are such effects relevant to the therapeutic action? in Handbook of Depression and Anxiety. Edited by den Boer JA, Sitsen JMA. New York, Marcel Dekker, 1994, pp 379–404

Lerer B, Stanley M: Does lithium stabilize muscarinic receptors? Biol Psychiatry 20:1247–1248, 1985

Li XM, Chlan-Fourney J, Juorio AV, et al: Antidepressants upregulate messenger RNA levels of the neuroprotective enzyme superoxide dismutase (SOD1). J Psychiatry Neurosci 25:43–47, 2000

Maier W, Lichtermann D, Minges J, et al: The relationship between bipolar disorder and alcoholism: a controlled family study. Psychol Med 25:787–796, 1995

Manji HK, Bebchuk JM, Moore GJ, et al: Modulation of CNS signal transduction pathways and gene expression by mood-stabilizing agents: therapeutic implications. J Clin Psychiatry 60 (suppl 2):27–39, 1999

Mann JJ, Malone KM: Cerebrospinal fluid amines and higher-lethality suicide attempts in depressed inpatients. Biol Psychiatry 41 (2):162–171, 1997

Mann JJ, Arango V, Marzuk PM: Evidence for the 5-HT hypothesis of suicide: a review of post-mortem studies. Br J Psychiatry 155 (suppl 8):7–14, 1989

Marangell LB, George MS, Callahan AM, et al: Effects of intrathecal thyrotropin-releasing hormone (protirelin) in refractory depressed patients. Arch Gen Psychiatry 54:214–222, 1997

Mathews R, Li PP, Young T, et al: Increased $G\alpha_{q/11}$ immunoreactivity in postmortem occipital cortex from patients with bipolar affective disorder. Biol Psychiatry 41:649–656, 1997

McBride PA, Brown RP, DeMeo M: The relationship of platelet 5-HT2 receptor indices to major depressive disorder, personality traits, and suicidal behavior. Biol Psychiatry 35:295–308, 1994

McKinney WT: Animal models for depression and mania, in Depression and Mania. Edited by Georgotas A, Cancro R. New York, Elsevier, 1988, pp 181–196

Okamoto Y, Kagaya A, Shinno H, et al: Serotonin-induced platelet calcium mobilization is enhanced in mania. Life Sci 56:327–332, 1995

Rush AJ, Giles DE, Schlesser MA, et al: Dexamethasone response, thyrotropin-releasing hormone stimulation, rapid eye movement latency, and subtypes of depression. Biol Psychiatry 41:915–928, 1997

Salomon RM, Miller HL, Krystal JH, et al: Lack of behavioral effects of monoamine depletion in healthy subjects. Biol Psychiatry 41:58–64, 1997

Schildkraut JJ: The catecholamine hypothesis of affective disorders: a review of supporting evidence. Am J Psychiatry 122:509–514, 1965

Schreiber G, Avissar S: G proteins as a biochemical tool for diagnosis and monitoring treatments of mental disorders. Isr Med Assoc J 2 (suppl): 86–91, 2000

Seligman MEP: Helplessness: On Depression, Development and Death. San Francisco, CA, WH Freeman, 1975

Serretti A, Lilli R, Lorenzi C, et al: Serotonin-2C and serotonin-1A receptor genes are not associated with psychotic symptomatology of mood disorders. Am J Med Genet 96:161–166, 2000

Siever LJ, Davis KL: Overview: toward a dysregulation hypothesis of depression. Am J Psychiatry 142:1017–1025, 1985

Soares JC, Mann JJ: The anatomy of mood disorders—review of structural neuroimaging studies. Biol Psychiatry 41:86–106, 1997

Stancer HC, Persad E: Treatment of intractable rapid-cycling manic-depressive disorder with levothyroxine: clinical observations. Arch Gen Psychiatry 39:311–312, 1982

Thase ME, Kupfer DJ, Fasiczka AJ, et al: Identifying an abnormal electroencephalographic sleep profile to characterize major depressive disorder. Biol Psychiatry 41:964–973, 1997

Tsuang MT, Faraone SV: The inheritance of mood disorders, in Genetics and Mental Illness: Evolving Issues for Research and Society. Edited by Hall LL. New York, Plenum, 1996, pp 79–109

Vallada H, Craddock N, Vasquez L, et al: Linkage studies in bipolar affective disorder with markers on chromosome 21. J Affect Disord 41:217–221, 1996

van Praag HM: Two-tier diagnosing in psychiatry. Psychiatry Res 34:1–11, 1990

Vawter MP, Freed WJ, Kleinman JE: Neuropathology of bipolar disorder. Biol Psychiatry 48:486–504, 2000

Whybrow PC, Akiskal HS, McKinney WJ: Mood Disorders: Toward a New Psychobiology. New York, Plenum, 1984, pp 21–42

Wirz-Justice A, Quinto C, Cajochen C, et al: A rapid-cycling bipolar patient treated with long nights, bedrest, and light. Biol Psychiatry 45:1075–1077, 1999

Woods BT, Yurgelun-Todd D, Mikulis D, et al: Age-related MRI abnormalities in bipolar illness: a clinical study. Biol Psychiatry 38:846–847, 1995

3

COURSE OF MOOD DISORDERS

All mood disorders are characterized by recurrence and chronicity. Although there is a good deal of support for the natural history of mood disorders, the psychobiology of progression is just beginning to be understood.

■ UNIPOLAR DEPRESSION

The mean age at onset of unipolar depression is 25–35 years. About 25% of patients have low-grade chronic or intermittent depression before experiencing a major depressive episode. When early studies showed that the depression of an increasing number of patients remitted during extended follow-up, it was concluded that most patients would eventually recover from a major depressive episode; however, longer studies have disproved this assumption. There is a 50% chance of remission of depression that has been present for 3–6 months, but there is only a 5% likelihood of remission, within the next 6 months, of a major depressive episode that has been present for 2 years (Keller et al. 1996). The same research suggests that about 12% of patients with acute major depression do not recover after 5 years of illness; 7% of those studied did not recover after 10 years (Keller et al. 1996).

Relapse, or the return before recovery of symptoms that meet criteria for a diagnosis of a disorder, implies a return of the index episode. *Recurrence,* which is a return of the disorder that develops after recovery, is considered a new episode. DSM-IV-TR (American Psychiatric Association 2000) defines *partial remission* as response with some persistent symptoms but not enough to meet criteria for major depression (or response with no symptoms) and lasting less than 2 months. Most experts consider persistence of anything more than minimal symptoms to be partial remission. Rates of partial remission in studies of antidepressants, psychotherapy, and/or behavior therapy have ranged from 4.9% to 42%.

Prospective follow-up studies continuing 2–20 years after an index major depressive episode suggest that 5%–27% (mean, 17%) of patients with major depressive disorder (MDD) remain chronically ill. In longitudinal investigations, about one-third of depressed patients are ill at any time. In DSM-IV-TR, recurrent and chronic MDD are diagnosed as recurrent major depression with full interepisode recovery and no dysthymia, recurrent major depressive episode without full interepisode recovery (i.e., residual major depression) but with no dysthymia, recurrent major depressive episode with full interepisode recovery but superimposed on dysthymia (double depression), and recurrent major depressive episode without full interepisode recovery, superimposed on dysthymia. After initial improvement, relapse may be followed by chronicity. However, these categories represent only some of the courses that unipolar mood disorders may follow.

In the National Institute of Mental Health Collaborative Study of the Psychobiology of Depression (NIMH-CS), 54% of patients with major unipolar depression recovered within the first 6 months of entry into the study, whereas only 18% of those who were still depressed after a year recovered between that time and the fifth year of this naturalistic study (Keller 1994). In a study involving subjects selected for an episodic course of major depression, Coryell and associates (1994) found that patients who did not recover from an episode within 2 months had a one-in-three chance of recovery over the next 2 months. The odds of recovery in any 2 of the next 8 months decreased to one in five to six. In the second year of depression, the likelihood of recovery in any 2-month period decreased to a little more than 7%. Such results confirm data just presented demonstrating that the longer major depression has been present, the more likely it is to persist. On the other hand, even patients who have been depressed for many years may eventually recover.

In the Zurich Study, 12%–14% of patients had a chronic course, which was defined as a Global Assessment Scale score of less than 61, a depression duration of at least 2 years, and no recovery over 5 years (Angst and Wicki 1991). In three other large studies in which patients were followed for 11–27 years, the rate of chronicity was 11%–25% (Angst and Wicki 1991). Predictors of a chronic course that emerged in these studies include psychosis, multiple losses, comorbid medical illness, substance dependence, a disabled spouse, agitation, anxiety, delusions, passive dependent or avoidant personality style, work impairment, double depression, and a family history of mood disorder or psychosis.

Major depressive episodes have a tendency to recur, even with treatment. In the NIMH-CS, 25% of patients who recovered during the first year relapsed within 3 months (Keller 1994). The rates of recurrence after recovery from an episode of major depression have been found to range from 50% within 2 years to 90% in 6 years (Coryell et al. 1994). After having been depressed once, the average person has at least a 50% chance of becoming depressed again, but after two episodes the risk of a third episode is 70%. After the third episode the risk of a fourth is 80%, and after four episodes the risk of another one is 90%. Overall, between 75% and 95% of patients who have experienced a major depressive episode will have at least one more episode over the course of their lives. On average, major depressive episodes recur every 5 years, the latency between episodes shortening from an average of 6 years after two episodes to just 2 years after three episodes. Around 15% of patients with unipolar depression have only one episode of major depression, whereas 13%–54% (mean, 27%) have three or more episodes. The average lifetime number of episodes of unipolar depression is four. The recurrence rates of both major depression and dysthymia are higher in double depression than in episodic MDD or dysthymic disorder without MDD. In the NIMH-CS, 4% of patients with episodic MDD experienced a relapse of an index major depressive episode within the first month of recovery, compared with 30% of patients with double depression (Keller 1994).

A number of factors have been found to increase the risk of relapse and recurrence of unipolar depression (Conte and Karasu 1992). One of the most important of these is inadequate treatment. Because residual depressive symptoms increase the risk of a relapse fourfold, any depressive episode should be treated as completely as possible. Persistent subthreshold symptoms (e.g., trouble concentrating, feelings of worthlessness, sleep disturbance, decreased sex drive, anxiety, impaired work, decreased initiative, and social maladjustment) are particularly important to recognize because they increase the risk of relapse and recurrence. Residual symptoms may have been present before the acute episode but may have been overshadowed by more florid acute symptoms. Persistence of these symptoms amounts to persistence of prodromal symptoms that will predict the next episode.

It can be difficult to determine whether periodic drops in mood indicate a partial antidepressant response or whether they represent nonclinical fluctuations in mood that do not predict relapse. One distinction between normal "blips" and partial or subclinical symptoms of relapse is that partial relapse symptoms are similar to those of the previous episode and tend to worsen over time, whereas nonclinical mood swings do not progress and are not similar to symptoms of previous depressive episodes.

To minimize the negative effect of residual symptoms on the course of mood disorders, it is important to use the most aggressive treatment possible, so that a remission rather than merely a response is produced. Psychotherapeutic treatment of residual psychological symptoms such as negative cognitions reduces the risk of recurrence after drug discontinuation (see Chapter 5). By the same token, discontinuation of effective treatment often leads to relapse, especially if medications are withdrawn rapidly or if even subtle residual symptoms or role dysfunction is present. A greater number of previous recurrences increases the risk. High expressed emotion in the family, marital problems, and psychosis also increase the risk of a relapse of unipolar depression. Secondary depression, whether associated with medical or nonaffective psychiatric illness, increases the risk of relapse by 60% and reduces the length of time to relapse. The severity of a depressive episode does not affect the risk of relapse.

In two 16-year follow-up studies involving hospitalized depressed patients, only 18%–20% recovered and were continuously well (Paykel 1982). Another 63% recovered, but these patients had subsequent episodes, and 17%–19% were continuously ill or committed suicide. Keller (1994) estimated that there is only a 22% chance of sustaining a recovery from major unipolar depression. In a review of published outcome studies, Piccinelli and Wilkinson (1994) noted that even though 90% of patients were found to have had remissions during 5 years of follow-up, only 24% of patients remained well for 10 years after an index episode. Maj et al. (1992) reported that 25% of patients remained well 5 years after recovering from an index major depressive episode. In a 20-year investigation, Angst (1998) found that patients who had an index episode of major depression spent an average of 20% of their lives in depressive episodes. In the NIMH-CS, one-third of 495 patients who were followed for 10 years after an index major depressive episode were in an episode at any point during the follow-up (Keller 1994).

A prospective 5-year follow-up study involving 86 outpatients with early-onset dysthymic disorder found that only 53% had recovered at the end of the study (Klein et al. 2000). Of those who recovered, 45% relapsed within 23 months, and for 70% of the follow-up period the sample met full criteria for a mood disorder. Of the patients who had never had a major depressive episode before study entry, 77% had a major depressive episode during follow-up.

In the National Institute of Mental Health Collaborative Depression Study, rates of recovery from a recurrence were similar to recovery rates after an index episode (Mueller and Leon 1996). In this particular investigation, each time a patient had another episode, there was an 8% chance of not recovering from that episode after 5 years. Preventing recurrence is therefore an important step toward reducing the accumulating risk of chronicity. Some clinicians prefer to wait before instituting treatment for a recurrence of unipolar depression, to see whether the recurrence will resolve rapidly. However, survival curves are similar for index and recurrent episodes. A recurrence therefore is not any more likely to remit spontaneously than a first episode, and rapid reintroduction of an antidepressant results in a response that is as prompt as the response to previous episodes.

■ BIPOLAR DISORDER

On average, the onset of bipolar disorder is 6 years earlier than that of unipolar depression, usually occurring by the second or third decade of life. However, first episodes of mania have been reported after age 50 years. The median duration of a manic episode is 5–10 weeks and that of a bipolar depressive episode is 19 weeks. Mixed bipolar episodes have a median duration of 36 weeks. Kraepelin distinguished between "manic-depressive insanity" and dementia praecox on the grounds that the former was characterized by complete remission between episodes and lack of deterioration. However, less than one-third of patients with acute bipolar affective episodes remain euthymic for a year, and 20% of acute affective episodes in bipolar disorder become chronic, with the highest rate of chronicity occurring in mixed bipolar episodes.

In patients with bipolar I disorder, the polarity of the initial episode predicts the polarity of the majority of subsequent episodes. In a retrospective study involving 320 patients with bipolar I disorder, 50% of first episodes were depressive (Perugi et al. 2000). Patients with an index depressive episode were more likely to develop rapid cycling, possibly as a result of early institution of antidepressant therapy, but they were less likely to develop psychosis. Patients with a mixed index episode were less likely to develop rapid cycling and more likely to have chronic mixed symptoms.

In patients who experience discrete recurrences of bipolar affective episodes, cycle length shortens during the first 3–6 episodes and then stabilizes at 1–2 episodes per year, the frequency of depressive and manic recurrences being about the same. The average patient with a bipolar mood disorder begins experiencing symptoms in adolescence and has had 10 or more acute affective episodes before age 35. Residual hypomanic symptoms increase the risk of depressive recurrences in bipolar mood disorder even more than do residual depressive symptoms. As with unipolar depression, the risk of bipolar relapse or recurrence decreases the longer a patient remains completely well (Coryell et al. 1994; Keller 1994). Likewise, starting treatment with mood-stabilizing medications earlier in the course of illness is associated with better prevention of recurrences than starting such treatment later in the course of illness.

The possible role of antidepressants in accelerating bipolar recurrences has been the subject of a good deal of debate. Antidepressants could contribute to rapid cycling by inducing mania or by speeding up the inherent cyclicity of bipolar mood disorders. However, although the majority of patients with rapid-cycling bipolar disorder are taking antidepressants, it is difficult to prove that antidepressants are the cause of rapid cycling. Alternative explanations would be that antidepressants are administered more frequently to patients with rapid-cycling and other forms of deteriorating bipolar disorder because depression is prominent or because nothing else is helping, or that rapid cycling would have developed with or without the use of an antidepressant. If assessment of the association between starting antidepressant therapy and the onset of rapid cycling is retrospective, the results are subject to being skewed by state-dependent recall and difficulty remembering the exact onset of complex mood swings. The only way to prove a causal relationship would be to follow prospectively matched patients with non-rapid-cycling bipolar mood disorder who had been randomly assigned to antidepressants or placebo, an experiment that is too difficult technically and ethically to be performed. Even in a prospective study, it is difficult to be certain whether rapid cycling that develops after months or years of treatment with an antidepressant has been caused by the medication.

These issues were addressed to some extent by Altshuler and associates (1995), who defined antidepressant-induced mania and rapid cycling as a first episode of severe mania or cycling appearing within 8 weeks of starting antidepressant therapy. In a literature review, the authors identified 158 patients with bipolar depression among patients with presumed unipolar depression who entered 15 placebo-controlled antidepressant trials. Thirty-five percent of patients in this subgroup likely met the stringent criterion for antidepressant-induced mania, the risk being more than 2.5 times as great (72% vs. 28%) among patients who were not also taking lithium. Inclusion of patients whose depression was obviously bipolar to begin with might have resulted in a different estimate.

Altshuler and her colleagues (1995) then used a life-chart method to characterize affective episodes in 51 patients with bipolar mood disorders refractory to lithium therapy; 55% of these patients had rapid cycling. Although 82% of the sample developed mania while taking antidepressants, the investigators concluded that only one-third met their criterion for antidepressant-induced mania. One reason for this low rate may have been that the patients had such a high rate of spontaneous affective episodes, and so many had taken antidepressants at some point, that it was not possible to detect increases attributable to an antidepressant. The authors found that antidepressant-induced mania increased the risk of rapid cycling by 4.6-fold. On the basis of their study and literature review, the authors suggested that the natural history of bipolar disorder and taking antidepressants each contributed to about 50% of the variance in the increased risk of rapid cycling, but withdrawing the antidepressant did not necessarily stop cycling. Most ominously, antimanic drugs did not predictably prevent or treat rapid cycling. In an earlier review of cases of refractory bipolar disorder, in which a similar methodology was used, mania was thought to be attributable to antidepressant therapy in 35% of patients and to rapid cycling in 26% (Roy-Byrne et al. 1985).

These results must be considered conservative for several reasons. First, hypomania and subsyndromal elevated mood were not included. Second, only classically defined rapid cycling was taken into account; other forms of mood cycling may be even more common and may be more or less prone than classic rapid cycling to being induced by antidepressants. The requirement that mania or mood cycling occur so soon after starting treatment with an antidepressant may have reduced the number of false-positive results, but it may have increased the likelihood of a type II error. Clinical experience suggests that there are a significant number of patients, especially those with ultradian (ultrarapid) cycling, whose moods become destabilized only after months to years of antidepressant therapy and whose depression and mood cycling are aggravated rather than ameliorated by antidepressants.

■ FUNCTIONAL OUTCOME

Functional outcome in depression is as poor as in chronic medical disorders such as diabetes mellitus and cardiovascular disease (Mueller and Leon 1996). In the prospective study of the Iowa 500, 17% of depressed patients were unable to work because of depression, and 22% had incapacitating symptoms (Mueller and Leon 1996). The medical outcomes study involving 22,462 outpatients in a health maintenance organization found that those with depressive disorders functioned more poorly in almost all areas measured than did patients with diabetes, cardiovascular disease, arthritis, or pulmonary disease (Mueller and Leon 1996). Similarly, in the NIMH-CS study, depressed patients compared with control subjects were less likely to be employed, earned less money, were more likely never to have been married, had poorer marital relationships if they were married, and were less satisfied with sexual activity, even if they were not clinically ill (Mueller and Leon 1996).

Social maladjustment persists for months after symptomatic remission of depression. If recovery is defined as the absence of disability and dysfunction as well as the absence of symptoms, many patients enrolled in clinical trials who are judged to be well symptomatically have had at best partial remissions of the entire illness. Symptoms and impairment of work, social, and parental roles often persist after improvement of depression, perhaps more frequently in double depression than in episodic MDD. Stewart et al. (1993) found that only 28% of patients with double depression who showed marked symptomatic improvement with treatment rated themselves as being well. Refractory major depression is associated with an increased risk of suicide, a 50% chance of work impairment, and a 65% risk of ongoing interpersonal distress. The risk of accidental death as well as of suicide is increased among all depressed patients (Mueller and Leon 1996). Compared with control subjects, depressed children are more impaired in mother–child interactions, peer relationships, and achievement and have more behavioral problems; impaired relationships may persist after symptomatic remission of depression.

These kinds of findings have important therapeutic implications. If mood disorders are defined only by their symptoms, treatment might be considered complete once specific symptoms have remitted. However, if role functioning, relationships, or overall health status is impaired, the mood disorder may still be active. In this case, further treatment might be considered, to reduce the risk of relapse even though the patient might not feel symptomatically ill.

■ CAUSES OF PROGRESSION OF MOOD DISORDERS

Mood disorders are not static but are dynamic conditions in which each new episode is a function of previous episodes, with an evolving course and treatment response. The evolution of these illnesses (the evolution of bipolar disorders is illustrated in Figure 3–1) is the result of an incompletely understood interaction among genetics, personality traits, environmental factors, cell biology, and, at times, medication and substance use (Post 1992). In many cases, initial episodes appear in response to an external stress, usually a loss or separation, or an event that evokes strong arousal or helplessness. The degree to which such events provoke an affective episode depends on their intrinsic severity and on predisposing and protective factors within the individual who experiences them. Mood in early episodes is often more reactive to the environment. Symptoms are less complex, and psychosocial disruption is less pervasive. A single

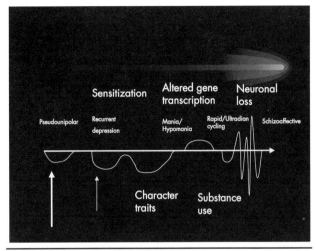

FIGURE 3–1. **Evolution of bipolar disorders.**

treatment is often effective, and the physiology as well as the psychology of abnormal mood remits completely with treatment in the absence of substantial genetic loading or overwhelming early adverse experience, indicating that the neurobiology of an initial affective episode is less complex. If they are not too severe, early depressive episodes respond equally well to environmental manipulation, psychotherapy, and medications. Early, uncomplicated hypomanic or even manic episodes may respond fully to a single antimanic drug or normalization of circadian rhythms.

As more affective episodes occur, the psychobiology of mood disorders appears to become more complex, with more spontaneous, frequent, and complex episodes and less euthymia. Sensitization of neuronal systems that mediate behavior and mood may be one factor in this evolution (Huber et al. 2001). At the same time, negative thinking, intrusiveness, arrogance, withdrawal, social ineptitude, irritability, and other depressive or manic behaviors elicit negative input from others, which reinforces feelings of helplessness and solidifies the patient's identity as someone who is unful-filled, overwhelmed, unpredictable, impulsive, incompetent, or unreliable. As more time is spent in periods of abnormal mood, re-missions are less complete and recurrences develop with less prov-ocation. These episodes are more likely to cause losses than to be caused by them.

In the case of bipolar disorder, sensitization of affective sys-tems with resetting of synaptic connections, and changes in gene expression induced by neurotransmitter, receptor, and second mes-senger responses to abnormal moods, may lead to nonlinear pro-gression and unpredictable alternations between inhibitory and excitatory influences on mood that might contribute to unstable mood cycling (Huber et al. 2001). Because rapid cycling seems more likely to develop after an episode of mania or hypomania, these states may be better sensitizing stimuli than depression. The ability of carbamazepine but not lithium to prevent kindling and be-havioral sensitization (D'Aquila et al. 2001) could explain why an-ticonvulsants such as carbamazepine are more effective than lithium for rapid cycling. The observation that imipramine induces supersensitivity to the locomotor effect of the dopamine D_2 receptor (D'Aquila et al. 2001) suggests that the contribution of antidepres-sant therapy to the development of rapid cycling may be related to behavioral sensitization as well as induction of mania.

Additional pressure on abnormal systems comes from sub-stances that can elicit affective dysregulation, especially those with stimulating, antidepressant, and psychotogenic effects such as co-caine and amphetamines. Environmental manipulations are not as successful at this point because the mood disorder is less responsive to external events. Psychological constellations are less amenable to structured psychotherapies and require more vigorous efforts to be-come reorganized. In cases in which administration of a single med-ication was initially effective, more complex interventions are necessary to address multiple interacting elements of abnormal cel-lular function. New medications aimed at second messengers or gene expression may prove useful for treating later-stage mood disorders involving multiple transmitter and receptor systems, and more aggressive and extended forms of psychotherapy may be necessary for mood disorders that have become integrated into the personality.

One feature of the progression of both unipolar and bipolar mood disorders is that cognitive dysfunction increasingly becomes a component of the illness. This aspect of the progression of mood disorders, an aspect that probably interacts with the aging process, may be a function of the very stress response that is inherent to mood disorders. Hypersecretion of corticotropin-releasing factor, which seems to be the proximate cause of hypercortisolemia in mood disorders, may be caused in part by inadequate negative feedback from the hippocampus, which also plays a critical role in learning, declarative memory, emotional processing, and development of adaptive responses to stress. Excessive concentrations of cortisol appear to cause both neuronal loss and dysfunction of remaining cells in the hippocampus, producing a level of cognitive impairment in both unipolar and bipolar mood disorders similar to that seen in Cushing's disease and syndromes caused by excessive exogenous corticosteroid therapy (Brown et al. 1999). An excessive stress response that may initially reflect an interaction among deficiencies in psychological adaptability, social support, and emotional regulation then further impairs the individual's problem-solving ability by damaging parts of the brain that are necessary to organize adaptive responses to future challenges (Figure 3–2).

The progression of bipolar mood disorders from more organized to more unstable and unpredictable states that become unresponsive to normal events and treatments is analogous to processes that have been described in other progressive medical disorders, such as cancer (see Figure 3–3). For example, progression of breast cancer is associated with mutations of the *BRCA1* and *BRCA2* susceptibility genes as well as induction of oncogenes and suppression of apoptotic genes (Loman et al. 2001). Mutations and changes in function of receptors such as the estrogen receptor that normally require extracellular growth factors (e.g., estrogen) to stimulate cellular proliferation make these receptors independent of normal homeostatic signals, which in turn makes treatments that block receptors ineffective (Talapatra and Thompson 2001).

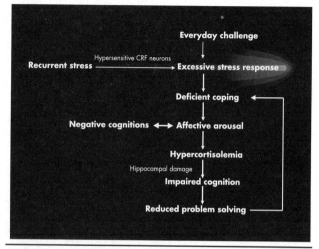

FIGURE 3–2. **Hippocampal damage by the stress response further impairs the stress response.**
Abbreviation: CRF=corticotropin-releasing factor.

With evolution from preinvasive to invasive to more poorly differentiated and independent of normal regulators of cell growth, tissue from many types of malignancies contains a growing number of genes that are abnormally expressed (Welsh et al. 2001). Some of these genes are disease specific, and some seem to be associated with progression of different cancers (Welsh et al. 2001). Loss of regulation of the *p53* tumor suppressor genes or the *ras* genes through mutation or errors of replication, for instance, lead to loss of regulation of other genes, the products of which are involved in cell cycle regulation, apoptosis, and DNA repair and are associated with uncontrolled proliferation, development of multiple tumors, and resistance to chemotherapy in cancers as diverse as leukemia, melanoma, osteosarcoma, breast cancer, ovarian cancer, and testicular cancer (Keshelava et al. 2001). The gene for the β_2 retinoic acid receptor, which is induced by chemotherapy with retinoids, is

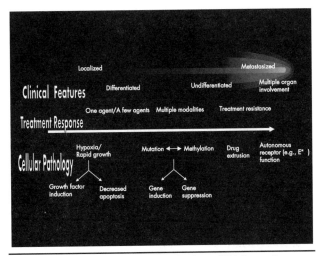

FIGURE 3–3. **Progressive changes in the cell biology of cancer.**

abnormally methylated in later stages of diseases such as breast cancer, leading to reduced or even absent expression and loss of response to retinoids (Widschwendter et al. 2001). Such epigenetic processes seem to be mediated both by treatment itself and by the disease process, as when hypoxia within rapidly growing cells induces genes that promote growth of blood vessels into the tumor as well as tumor cell growth. Alteration of the structure of regulatory genes as the treatment interacts with the illness creates a new disease that is more complex and more refractory to treatment.

Just as some cases of cancer perpetuate themselves and become more complex through alterations of gene expression and the function of regulatory processes, some cases of bipolar disorder have the capacity to accelerate, probably through multiple changes in synaptic regulation that in all likelihood result from alterations of multiple gene products stimulated by the disease process, possibly through interaction with some treatments. Because there are many sources of input to the functioning of neurotransmitters, receptors, second messengers, and other intracellular processes that together constitute the neuronal "thymostat," different changes in gene expression induced by experience, treatment, and the mood disorder itself can produce similar phenotypes of deteriorating mood. This situation is also directly analogous to cancer, in which patients with similar histologies have different patterns of gene expression, different family histories, and different treatment responses (Loman et al. 2001).

The possibility that mood-stabilizing medications may normalize intracellular signaling and gene expression is suggested by evidence that lithium and carbamazepine have calcium antagonist properties and regulate calcium-dependent intracellular proteins such as protein kinase C; lithium and valproate alter expression of the glucose-regulated protein 78 gene, DNA regulator proteins such as activator protein-1 (AP-1), and intracellular neuroprotective proteins such as N-acetyl aspartate and Bcl-2; lamotrigine inhibits glutamate release and calcium influx; and antimanic drugs as diverse in structure as valproate and lithium inhibit protein kinase C in addition to altering expression of the AP-1 family of transcription factors and of a reporter gene driven by an AP-1 promoter (Dubovsky et al. 1992; Manji et al. 1999; Wang et al. 2001). Obviously, the mechanism of action of treatments for mood disorders goes beyond single neurotransmitter or receptor systems and even beyond single second messengers. Different actions on different intracellular systems may explain why one medication is more effective than another for a given patient. The more that is understood about the evolution of intracellular pathology in mood disorders, the better able researchers and clinicians will be to develop specific treatments for these conditions and to prevent the interactions between illness and treatment that lead to treatment resistance.

■ REFERENCES

Altshuler LL, Post RM, Leverich GS: Antidepressant-induced mania and cycle acceleration: a controversy revisited. Am J Psychiatry 152:1130–1138, 1995

American Psychiatric Association: Diagnostic and Statistical Manual of Mental Disorders, 4th Edition, Text Revision. Washington, DC, American Psychiatric Association, 2000

Angst J: Clinical course of affective disorders, in Depressive Illness: Prediction of Course and Outcome. Edited by Hedgsort T, Daly RJ. Berlin, Germany, Springer, 1998, pp 205–250

Angst J, Wicki W: The Zurich Study, XI: is dysthymia a separate form of depression? Results of the Zurich Cohort Study. Eur Arch Psychiatry Clin Neurosci 240:349–354, 1991

Barnet PW, Harrison PJ: Substance P (NK1) receptors in the cingulate cortex in unipolar and bipolar mood disorder and schizophrenia. Biol Psychiatry 47:80–83, 2000

Brown ES, Rush AJ, McEwen BS: Hippocampal remodeling and damage by corticosteroids: implications for mood disorders. Neuropsychopharmacology 21:474–484, 1999

Conte HR, Karasu TB: A review of treatment studies of minor depression: 1980–1991. Am J Psychother 46:58–74, 1992

Coryell W, Akiskal HS, Leon AC, et al: The time course of nonchronic major depressive disorder. Arch Gen Psychiatry 51:405–410, 1994

D'Aquila PS, Peana AT, Tanda O, et al: Carbamazepine prevents imipramine-induced behavioural sensitization to the dopamine D(2)-like receptor agonist quinpirole. Eur J Pharmacol 416:107–111, 2001

DeVane CL: Substance P: a new era, a new role. Pharmacotherapy 21:1061–1069, 2001

Dubovsky SL, Murphy J, Christiano J, et al: The calcium second messenger system in bipolar disorders: data supporting new research directions. J Neuropsychiatry Clin Neurosci 4:3–14, 1992

Huber MT, Braun HA, Krieg JC: On the impact of episode sensitization on the course of recurrent affective disorders. J Psychiatr Res 35:49–57, 2001

Keller MB: Dysthymia in clinical practice: course, outcome and impact on the community. Acta Psychiatr Scand Suppl 383:24–34, 1994

Keller MB, Hanks DL, Klein DN: Summary of the DSM-IV mood disorders field trial and issue overview. Psychiatr Clin North Am 19:1–27, 1996

Keshelava N, Zao JJ, Chen P, et al: Loss of *p53* function confers high level multidrug resistance in neuroblastoma cell lines. Cancer Res 61:6185–6195, 2001

Klein DN, Schwartz JE, Rose S, et al: Five-year course and outcome of dysthymic disorder: a prospective, naturalistic follow-up study. Am J Psychiatry 157:931–939, 2000

Loman N, Johannsson O, Kristoffersson U, et al: Family history of breast and ovarian cancers and *BRCA1* and *BRCA2* mutations in a population-based series of early onset breast cancer. J Natl Cancer Inst 93:1215–1223, 2001

Maj M, Veltro F, Pirozzi R, et al: Pattern of recurrence of illness after recovery from an episode of major depression: a prospective study. Am J Psychiatry 149:795–800, 1992

Manji HK, Bebchuk JM, Moore GJ, et al: Modulation of CNS signal transduction pathways and gene expression by mood-stabilizing agents: therapeutic implications. J Clin Psychiatry 60 (suppl 2):27–39, 1999

Mueller TI, Leon AC: Recovery, chronicity, and levels of psychopathology in major depression. Psychiatr Clin North Am 19:85–102, 1996

Paykel ES: Handbook of Affective Disorders. New York, Guilford, 1982

Perugi G, Micheli C, Akiskal HS, et al: Polarity of the first episode, clinical characteristics, and course of manic depressive illness: a systematic retrospective investigation of 320 bipolar I patients. J Clin Psychiatry 41:13–18, 2000

Piccinelli M, Wilkinson G: Outcome of depression in psychiatric settings. Br J Psychiatry 164:297–304, 1994

Post RM: Transduction of psychosocial stress into the neurobiology of recurrent affective disorder. Am J Psychiatry 149:999–1010, 1992

Roy-Byrne P, Post RM, Uhde TW, et al: The longitudinal course of recurrent affective illness: life chart data from research patients at the NIMH. Acta Psychiatr Scand Suppl 317:1–34, 1985

Stewart JW, McGrath PJ, Quitkin FM: Chronic depression: response to placebo, imipramine, and phenelzine. J Clin Psychopharmacol 13:391–396, 1993

Talapatra S, Thompson CB: Growth factor signaling in cell survival: implications for cancer treatment. J Pharmacol Exp Ther 298:873–878, 2001

Wang JF, Bown CD, Chen B, et al: Identification of mood stabilizer-regulated genes by differential-display PCR. Int J Neuropsychopharmacol 4:65–74, 2001

Welsh JB, Sapinoso LM, Su AI, et al: Analysis of gene expression identifies candidate markers and pharmacological targets in prostate cancer. Cancer Res 61:5974–5978, 2001

Widschwendter M, Berger J, Muller HM, et al: Epigenetic downregulation of the retinoic acid receptor-beta2 gene in breast cancer. J Mammary Gland Biol Neoplasia 6:193–201, 2001

4

SOMATIC THERAPIES
FOR MOOD DISORDERS

In this brief review, we summarize essential aspects of the treatment of depression with medications and other physical therapies such as electroconvulsive therapy (ECT), bright light therapy, and repetitive transcranial magnetic stimulation (rTMS). We also discuss drugs and treatments used to stabilize mood in bipolar disorder. More comprehensive discussions of pharmacological therapies can be found in standard texts (e.g., Schatzberg and Nemeroff 1998).

■ TREATMENTS FOR DEPRESSION

Antidepressant Medications

Antidepressants are traditionally classified according to their structure (e.g., tricyclics, tetracyclics) or their effect on neurotransmitters (e.g., norepinephrine reuptake inhibitors, serotonin reuptake inhibitors, monoamine oxidase inhibitors [MAOIs]) or receptors (e.g., serotonin$_2$ [5-HT$_2$] antagonists). Although it is unlikely that any particular neurotransmitter action can account for the therapeutic effect of antidepressants, neurotransmitter actions do predict side effects. For example, noradrenergic antidepressants can produce jitteriness, tremor, sweating, and insomnia; serotonergic antidepressants cause nausea, headaches, and sexual dysfunction; and dopaminergic antidepressants are activating and can increase blood pressure.

All antidepressants are associated with about a 60% response rate in nonpsychotic unipolar depression, which is significantly higher than the 20%–40% response rate associated with placebo. Although antidepressants have been found to be effective for milder depression, the difference between active antidepressant and placebo diminishes as the severity of depression increases. The high placebo response rate (up to 50%–70%) in less severe forms of depression results in an overall effect size of only 0.5 in nonpsychotic, nonbipolar depression of mild to moderate severity (Doris et al. 1999).

A number of limitations of clinical trials make extrapolating results to clinical practice difficult. For example, the fact that the end point of most trials is response (i.e., 50% improvement) rather than remission inflates the benefit in a clinical trial, because most people would prefer not to settle for this level of improvement. The rate of remission after 8 weeks of treatment—longer than most clinical trials last—is only 30% (Burke and Preskhorn 1995). Studies required for U.S. Food and Drug Administration (FDA) approval need last only 4–6 weeks and do not provide information about long-term efficacy or adverse effects. In fact, a multicenter study involving 900 depressed patients treated with adequate doses of antidepressants found a time to remission in more than half the patients of more than 6 weeks, and the Treatment of Depression Collaborative Study (Elkin et al. 1989) found that even 16 weeks of treatment with antidepressants or psychotherapy were not enough to achieve full recovery and lasting remission.

The use in many trials of the method of analysis involving the last observation carried forward can also be problematic. In this method, the last measure obtained from patients who drop out is considered to be the final value for those patients. Patients who withdraw early from a clinical trial because of adverse effects or for some other reason may appear not to have responded, because the antidepressant has not yet had a chance to become effective; the apparent efficacy of the drug is thus artificially reduced in these patients. This problem is common in comparisons with older antidepressants (e.g., imipramine), which have adverse effects that frequently lead patients to discontinue them prematurely. In actual clinical settings, more attention is paid to providing support for medication continuation than in a placebo-controlled study, and the rate of response to active medication is often higher. Although considering patients who drop out because of adverse effects as not having responded to treatment may mirror clinical experience that a medication that patients cannot tolerate is for all intents and purposes ineffective, the use of fixed doses and a lack of opportunities to treat adverse effects or change medications can also lead to an underestimation of antidepressant efficacy in clinical trials.

Premarketing studies involve relatively brief trials and relatively small numbers of patients, typically 2,500 or fewer people, 90% of whom have been enrolled in Phase I or Phase II studies in which doses are different from those most commonly used in clinical practice (Burke and Preskhorn 1995). Phase III clinical trials often also use doses lower than those used in clinical practice, in order to minimize the number of dropouts due to adverse effects. Even so, 20%–40% of patients drop out of randomized clinical trials, and not enough is known about these patients to determine how data obtained from them might affect overall results. Patients selected for clinical trials usually are 18–65 years old and have relatively mild forms of depression without chronicity, comorbidity, or a history of treatment resistance, making them more similar to depressed patients treated by primary care physicians than to the more complex and severely ill patients treated by psychiatrists (Partonen et al. 1996). In accordance with FDA requirements, new antidepressants are usually compared with placebo rather than with other newer established antidepressants, which makes it difficult to know whether one new antidepressant is better than another in a particular situation. At the same time, in an attempt to recoup the $500 million it costs to bring a new antidepressant to the market (Burke and Preskhorn 1995), pharmaceutical manufacturers exploit minor differences that are not clinically meaningful, to encourage clinicians to prescribe their product.

Tricyclic and tetracyclic antidepressants (Table 4–1) have a three- or four-carbon-ring structure. All these medications have similar properties. In most cases, either the parent drugs (e.g., desipramine) or their metabolites (e.g., desmethylclomipramine) block

TABLE 4–1. Tricyclic and tetracyclic antidepressants

Generic name	Trade name	Usual daily dose (mg)	Comments
Amitriptyline	Elavil	150–300	Sedating, anticholinergic; metabolized to nortriptyline
Amoxapine	Asendin	150–600	A metabolite of loxapine, an antipsychotic; 7-OH metabolite of amoxapine has antipsychotic properties
Clomipramine	Anafranil	150–250	Only tricyclic effective for OCD; doses >250 mg/day can cause seizures
Desipramine	Norpramin, Pertofrane	150–300	Therapeutic window in some studies 125–200 ng/mL
Doxepin	Adapin, Sinequan	100–300	Like trimipramine; useful for treating allergies, esophagitis, peptic ulcer
Imipramine	Tofranil	150–300	Reference antidepressant; metabolized to desipramine
Maprotiline	Ludiomil	150–225	A tetracyclic between imipramine and desipramine in side-effect profile; doses >225 mg/day associated with increased risk of seizures
Nortriptyline	Aventyl, Pamelor	75–150	Therapeutic window 50–150 ng/mL
Protriptyline	Vivactil	15–60	Used for sleep apnea
Trimipramine	Surmontil	150–300	As potent as cimetidine as histamine H_1 receptor antagonist

Note. OCD=obsessive-compulsive disorder.

norepinephrine reuptake, and some parent drugs (e.g., chlorimipramine, imipramine) block 5-HT reuptake. Neurotransmitter reuptake inhibition mainly predicts adverse effects. For example, noradrenergic antidepressants are more likely to cause arousal, diaphoresis, tremor, anxiety, and insomnia, and serotonergic antidepressants are more likely to produce headaches, sedation, agitation, gastrointestinal side effects, and sexual dysfunction. However, clomipramine (chlorimipramine), which is a potent serotonin reuptake inhibitor, is the only tricyclic antidepressant (TCA) that is effective in the treatment of obsessive-compulsive disorder.

All TCAs have similar side-effect profiles (Glassman and Preud'homme 1993). A quinidine-like effect makes TCAs as effective as the type Ia antiarrhythmics in the treatment of ventricular tachyarrhythmias. For the same reason, these medications can aggravate heart block and have a negative inotropic effect. Tertiary amine TCAs such as imipramine and amitriptyline have more anticholinergic and sedative side effects than secondary amine TCAs such as desipramine and nortriptyline. The tertiary amines also produce more α_1-adrenergic blockade, resulting in postural hypotension, and produce more histamine H_1 antagonism, which contributes to sedation and weight gain. These kinds of adverse effects, along with the potential negative impact on memory of anticholinergic side effects, make the tertiary amine TCAs poor choices for older patients and patients with dementia. Nortriptyline and desipramine are better tolerated by older patients. As noted in Table 4–1, nortriptyline has a therapeutic window, and desipramine probably has a therapeutic window as well. Aside from a sinusoidal correlation between serum level and clinical response for imipramine and possibly amitriptyline, no other correlations between serum antidepressant level and clinical response have been demonstrated (Perry et al. 1994). Measuring antidepressant levels (i.e., therapeutic drug monitoring) may be useful mostly for determining whether nonresponse to a high antidepressant dose or adverse effects with a low dose may be due to unexpectedly low or high serum levels.

Second-generation antidepressants (Table 4–2) are heterogeneous with respect to their structures and actions. Trazodone is pri-

TABLE 4–2. Second- and third-generation antidepressants

Generic name	Trade name	Usual daily dose (mg)	Comments
Bupropion	Wellbutrin	200–450	Sustained-release preparation still requires twice-daily dosing; drug can be used to treat SSRI-induced sexual dysfunction.
Citalopram	Celexa	10–40	Minimal cytochrome P450 interactions but similar side effects compared with other SSRIs.
Escitalopram	Lexapro	10–20	S-enantiomer of citalopram has fewer adverse effects than citalopram, a finding that could be a function of doses half those of citalopram in comparisons with citalopram and placebo.
Fluoxetine	Prozac	10–60	Therapeutic window may develop over time, requiring reduction in dose; parent drug has half-life of 3 days; active metabolite has half-life of 6–9 days; fluoxetine can be more activating than other SSRIs.
Fluvoxamine	Luvox	100–300	Shorter half-life may necessitate twice-daily dosing.
Mirtazapine	Remeron	15–45	Could have antiemetic properties; oversedation and weight gain are common; best suited for older patients.
Nefazodone	Serzone	200–600	Useful for sleep disorders, fibromyalgia, chronic pain; divided dose usually necessary.
Paroxetine	Paxil	10–40	Anticholinergic properties equivalent to those of nortriptyline; more weight gain than with other SSRIs.
Sertraline	Zoloft	50–200	One metabolite with minimal activity.
Trazodone	Desyrel	200–600	Divided dose necessary for antidepressant effect.
Venlafaxine	Effexor	75–375	Effective for refractory depression; discontinuation syndrome can be troublesome.

Note. SSRI=selective serotonin reuptake inhibitor.

marily a 5-HT$_2$ receptor antagonist with prominent sedative properties. It is frequently used as a hypnotic because its short elimination half-life results in less daytime impairment than that caused by some traditional hypnotics. The same feature means that multiple doses of trazodone are necessary to maintain steady-state concentrations. However, daytime sedation may limit this schedule. In 1 in 6,000 patients taking trazodone, α_1-adrenergic blockade causes priapism, which can result in impotence if not treated promptly. This adverse effect is not dose related. Bupropion is not sedating and does not have anticholinergic, sexual, sedative, or cardiotoxic side effects. However, divided doses are necessary even with the sustained-release form, and doses greater than 450 mg/day are associated with a 5% incidence of seizures, which is a greater problem in bulimic patients.

Six serotonin reuptake inhibitors (fluoxetine, sertraline, paroxetine, fluvoxamine, citalopram, escitalopram; see Table 4–2) are available in the United States. Although these medications are often referred to as selective serotonin reuptake inhibitors (SSRIs), none is truly selective clinically or pharmacologically. In addition to being effective for major depression, the SSRIs have applications in anxiety disorders, obsessive-compulsive disorder, posttraumatic stress disorder, eating disorders, and other conditions associated with dysregulation of functions that are moderated by serotonergic systems, such as unpredictable, unprovoked aggression; recurrent, intrusive thinking; and excessive sexual or appetitive behavior. Although SSRIs are more effective at blocking in vitro reuptake of 5-HT than are other neurotransmitters, potency in serotonin reuptake inhibition does not parallel antidepressant potency, and tianeptine, a TCA discussed in Chapter 2, enhances 5-HT reuptake.

As stated earlier, SSRIs all have similar side effects, including nausea, diarrhea, headache, activation, sedation, and sexual dysfunction. Interactions between 5-HT and other neurotransmitters make an isolated action on 5-HT in the intact nervous system impossible, even if an SSRI is entirely selective for 5-HT reuptake in the laboratory. An action on 5-HT$_2$ heteroreceptors located on dopaminergic neurons in the basal ganglia can result in reduced dopaminergic transmission, which is sometimes manifested as emotional blunting and extrapyramidal side effects (Dubovsky and Thomas 1996). When the medication is otherwise well tolerated and effective, these side effects can be treated with dopaminergic agents such as bupropion or a stimulant. Although reports of worsening of Parkinson's disease with SSRI administration have been variable, a possible antidopaminergic effect makes SSRIs second-line agents for patients with this disorder. SSRIs can exacerbate hypoglycemia associated with treatment of diabetes mellitus; however, the incidence of weight gain is lower than with older antidepressants, and thus SSRIs are often used for patients with this disease or other medical illnesses. Paroxetine has been associated with an influenza-like syndrome, rebound depression on withdrawal, and a discontinuation syndrome characterized by cholinergic rebound. This medication also inhibits norepinephrine reuptake at high doses, but this action is probably not therapeutically important.

The use of SSRIs in patients with medical illnesses requires awareness of interactions with other medications. Some interactions with oxidative metabolism by cytochrome P450 (CYP) 2D6 and CYP 3A4 are listed in Tables 4–3 and 4–4. (A more complete discussion of the actions of antidepressants and other psychiatric medications with cytochrome P450 enzymes can be found in Cozza and Armstrong 2001.) Although sertraline is a weak inhibitor of 2D6, this interaction is not important clinically most of the time. Citalopram does not have clinically important cytochrome P450 interactions. Inhibitors of cytochrome P450 enzymes increase serum levels and prolong elimination half-lives of substrates of that enzyme, but actual clinical interactions are difficult to predict because most medications act on more than one enzyme, actions on other metabolizing enzymes may also occur, and individual differences exist in susceptibility of a particular enzyme to inhibition or induction. In addition, other cytochrome P450 enzymes are involved in the metabolism of psychiatric and medical drugs, as are completely different matabolic processes such as glucuronidation and the drug extrusion protein P-glycoprotein.

TABLE 4–3. **Some cytochrome P450 (CYP) 2D6 substrates and interactors**

Substrates	Inhibitors	Inducers
Antiarrhythmics	Fluoxetine	Carbamazepine
β-Blockers	Fluphenazine, haloperidol,	Erythromycin (mild)
Butyrophenones,	perphenazine, quinidine,	Ketoconazole (mild)
clozapine,	thioridazine	Phenytoin
phenothiazines,	Paroxetine	Quinidine
risperidone	Sertraline (mild)	Venlafaxine (mild)
Codeine (to morphine)		
Dextromethorphan		
Fluoxetine, paroxetine		
Neurotoxins		
Procarcinogens,		
?carcinogens		
TCAs		
Venlafaxine		

Note. TCA=tricyclic antidepressant.

One issue of controversy has been the possible clinical effects of inhibition of 2D6 on carcinogenesis. It was proposed that 2D6 inhibition by some SSRIs could inhibit metabolism of carcinogens, but because the same enzyme is responsible for conversion of procarcinogens to carcinogens, these medications could have the potential to reduce carcinogenesis. There is no evidence of a clinically important effect on cancer risk by any of these medications, but calcium channel–blocking agents (discussed in "Treatments for Bipolar Disorder," in the section entitled "Calcium Channel–Blocking Agents") are used to antagonize a cellular pump that extrudes cancer chemotherapy drugs, the induction of which is associated with treatment resistance of some cancers.

Several third-generation antidepressants act on various neurotransmitters and receptors, with or without serotonin reuptake inhibition. Treatment with venlafaxine—which inhibits reuptake of 5-HT alone at doses less than 150 mg/day, norepinephrine and 5-HT at higher doses, and, to a lesser extent, dopamine—has been

TABLE 4–4. **Some cytochrome P450 (CYP) 3A4 substrates and interactors**

Substrates	Inhibitors	Inducers
Acetaminophen, codeine	Diltiazem, verapamil	Carbamazepine
Carbamazepine, ethosuximide	Erythromycin	Phenobarbital
Clonazepam	Fluoxetine	Phenytoin
Cortisol, estrogen, progesterone	Fluvoxamine	
Cyclosporine	Grapefruit juice	
Digitalis	Ketoconazole	
Diltiazem, nifedipine, nimodipine, verapamil	Nefazodone	
Nonsedating antihistamines	Venlafaxine	
Sertraline, TCAs		
Tamoxifen		
Triazolobenzodiazepines		
Type IA antiarrhythmics		

Note.   TCA=tricyclic antidepressant.

found to be efficacious in refractory depression. The immediate-release form of venlafaxine requires divided dosing, which is also necessary with higher doses of the sustained-release form. Venlafaxine can have adverse effects related to all three neurotransmitters affected (e.g., sexual dysfunction, jitteriness, and hypertension). Mild increases in diastolic blood pressure can occur; more severe hypertension develops rarely. Rapid discontinuation of venlafaxine has been associated with withdrawal symptoms including headache, nausea, fatigue, dizziness, dysphoria, rebound depression, and occasionally hallucinations.

Nefazodone, another third-generation antidepressant, has serotonin reuptake inhibitor and 5-HT$_2$ antagonist properties that could make it useful for severe and psychotic depression. Unlike most antidepressants, nefazodone does not suppress rapid eye movement (REM) sleep, and therefore the drug is associated with a lower incidence of disturbing dreams caused by REM rebound. The sedative properties of nefazodone and the possible improvement of (or at least lack of interference with) slow-wave sleep make nefazodone a useful drug for treating patients with insomnia, but because of its short half-life, divided dosing is required, which can be difficult when patients experience daytime sedation or dizziness. A "black box" warning about possible hepatotoxicity, recently added by the FDA, is based on 18 cases of hepatotoxicity (one of them fatal) out of about 10 million patients who have taken the drug worldwide.

Mirtazapine, a third-generation antidepressant that is related to the antidepressant mianserin, is an antagonist of $5\text{-}HT_2$ and $5\text{-}HT_3$ receptors and norepinephrine presynaptic α_2-adrenergic receptors. Antagonism of $5\text{-}HT_2$ receptors could prove useful for treating psychotic depression, whereas $5\text{-}HT_3$ receptor blockade has an antiemetic effect. Mirtazapine is now supplied as a chewable tablet, making it useful for older and medically ill patients who have difficulty swallowing pills. Sedation and weight gain are common adverse effects of mirtazapine, but the same properties, along with the antiemetic effect, make mirtazapine a first-line agent for depressed cancer patients with nausea, weight loss, and/or insomnia.

Monoamine oxidase inhibitors (MAOIs; see Table 4–5) may be more frequently effective than TCAs for major depression with atypical features. SSRIs also appear to be more effective than TCAs for atypical depression, although possibly less effective than MAOIs. All MAOIs are administered in divided doses. Although side-effect profiles differ, all medications in this class have the potential to induce activation, which often leads to insomnia and which can sometimes mimic hypomania in patients without bipolar disorder.

The most important limitations on the use of MAOIs have been 1) hypertensive reactions when sympathomimetic medications are taken or foods high in tyramine are ingested and 2) serotonin syndrome when serotonergic substances such as SSRIs or dextromethorphan are used concurrently. These problems arise because inhibition of monoamine oxidase A (MAO A) in the small intestine as well as the brain leads to absorption of excessive amounts of tyramine, a pressor amine found in many foods that is metabolized by intestinal MAO A. Intestinal and systemic inhibition of monoamine oxidase lead to accumulation of toxic levels of 5-HT, which is also metabolized by monoamine oxidase.

TABLE 4–5. Monoamine oxidase inhibitors

Generic name	Trade name	Usual daily dose (mg)	Comments
Isocarboxazid	Marplan	10–60	Less activating
Phenelzine	Nardil	45–90	Commonly causes weight gain and has anticholinergic side effects
Selegiline	Eldepryl	20–50	Activating; may enhance cognition and slow CNS deterioration
Tranylcypromine	Parnate	30–80	More activating; amphetamine-like metabolite may interact with parent drug; weight gain sometimes occurs

Note. CNS=central nervous system.

Two approaches to minimizing this problem have emerged (Kato et al. 1998). The first involves developing medications that are selective for monoamine oxidase B, which is present in high concentrations in the brain but not the gastrointestinal tract. Selegiline is an example of a selective MAOI, but at antidepressant doses it loses its selectivity and dietary restrictions must be followed. The second approach is exemplified by the drug moclobemide, a reversible inhibitor of MAO A (RIMA) that is easily displaced from the enzyme by tyramine, allowing the tyramine to be metabolized normally. Moclobemide is available in a number of countries but not in the United States, because the manufacturer determined that the patent would expire before the cost of gaining FDA approval could be recovered. Other RIMAs have not yet been released.

Antipsychotic Medications

The likelihood of response of psychotic depression to a combination of an antipsychotic drug and an antidepressant is significantly greater than the chance of response to either one alone. Most research on the use of antipsychotic medications in psychotic unipolar depression has involved the antipsychotics, especially perphenazine. These studies suggest that to achieve remission of psychotic depression, it may be necessary for psychotics to be given at higher doses (e.g., >32 mg of perphenazine per day) than those used to treat schizophrenia. Particularly at higher doses, adverse effects of neuroleptics can be problematic. Akinesia can mimic depression, leading to unnecessary dose escalation. Nonschizophrenic patients may be more vulnerable to other adverse effects such as tardive dyskinesia. Withdrawal of the antipsychotic may lead to relapse of depression without psychosis, and withdrawal of the antidepressant may be followed by relapse of psychosis without depression. Thus, treatment of psychotic depression is not separate treatments of two different symptoms; rather, it involves integrated treatment of a complex syndrome.

Amoxapine, a TCA that is a metabolite of loxapine and has the potency of antipsychotics (25 mg of amoxapine is equivalent to about 1 mg of haloperidol), is the only antidepressant that has been found effective as a monotherapeutic agent for psychotic depression in a double-blind study; loxapine has also been noted to be effective for psychotic depression in open studies (Anton and Burch 1993). The obvious disadvantage of both these medications is that it is impossible to adjust the antipsychotic separately from the antidepressant. In addition, both medications can have neurological side effects, including tardive dyskinesia.

Because some psychotically depressed patients, especially those with mild or intermittent psychotic symptoms, may respond to an antidepressant, some clinicians begin treatment of psychotic depression with an antidepressant and add an antipsychotic drug if the patient does not respond. Patients who have been pretreated with an antidepressant respond to the addition of an antipsychotic within 2 weeks. Treatment for psychotically depressed patients with severe or pervasive psychotic symptoms and those who are agitated, self-destructive, or homicidal is begun with an antipsychotic drug, an antidepressant–antipsychotic drug combination, or ECT.

Because they are better tolerated than antipsychotics, atypical antipsychotic medications have an obvious potential advantage in the treatment of psychotic depression. An additional advantage is that these medications have repeatedly been demonstrated to have antidepressant properties that may be separate from their antipsychotic effect (Marder 1998). Although there are no published double-blind studies of atypical antipsychotic drugs as either single agents or adjuvant drugs in psychotic depression, the experience of many clinicians is that they are preferable to antipsychotics as first-line therapeutic agents. It is not yet known whether, as is sometimes true of antipsychotics, higher doses of these medications may be necessary, but in studies of schizophrenia, concomitant depressive symptoms are usually more reliably reduced at higher doses. Despite the lack of controlled data, there is enough clinical experience to warrant using an atypical antipsychotic medication before an antipsychotic.

There is a group of patients with severe nonpsychotic depression who respond to antidepressants as poorly as patients with psychotic depression (Kocsis et al. 1988). In an 8-week, double-blind, randomized trial involving 28 patients with recurrent nonpsychotic, nonbipolar depression that had been resistant to treatment with antidepressants, olanzapine or fluoxetine alone produced significantly less improvement than the combination of the two medications (Shelton et al. 2001b). Insufficient data about individual patients were reported to determine whether the results support the hypothesis discussed in the section on psychotic depression in Chapter 1 that dimensions of depression such as severity, cognitive dysfunction, dissociation, or recurrence that occur more frequently in psychotic depression may influence response to the addition of an antipsychotic drug to an antidepressant.

Electroconvulsive Therapy

ECT is the most effective treatment for bipolar and unipolar depression and the most rapidly effective treatment for mania (Dubovsky 1995). Animal studies indicate that ECT has an effect on G protein function that is similar to that of lithium (Avissar and Schreiber 1992).

In ECT, a bidirectional square wave lasting about 2 milliseconds is applied through right (nondominant) unilateral or bilateral electrodes to produce a generalized electrical seizure in the brain lasting 20–150 seconds. Although it was initially introduced as a treatment for schizophrenia, ECT is now known to benefit only about 15% of patients with this diagnosis—generally those with an acute illness of relatively brief duration accompanied by affective symptoms, perplexity, catatonia, and good premorbid adjustment. ECT is most clearly useful in the case of acute major depressive episodes, especially when they are characterized by rapid onset, brief duration, severity, psychosis, motor retardation, catatonia, severe pseudodementia, lack of insight, and inability to tolerate antidepressants (Dubovsky 1995). ECT is also highly effective in mania and catatonia. At one time, it was thought that ECT would be inappropriate in the presence of delirium because ECT induces an acute confusional state, but more recent experience has shown that ECT can produce rapid improvement in delirium. Motor symptoms of Parkinson's disease and the on–off phenomenon also improve with ECT, independent of ECT's effect on depressed mood (Dubovsky 1995). ECT has been found to be safe and effective in children as well as adults (Willoughby et al. 1997).

Evidence has emerged of a relationship between the dose of the electrical stimulus and response to ECT, at least in unipolar depression, in which stimulus intensities three times the seizure threshold appear to be more reliably effective. Right unilateral ECT is usually used first in the treatment of a major depressive episode because it is associated with a lower risk of cognitive impairment. Bilateral ECT is used in cases of nonresponse to unilateral ECT and as an initial approach in cases of severe depression, psychotic depression, catatonic stupor, Parkinson's disease, and depression in which a smaller number of ECT treatments is desirable (e.g., in cases of high anesthetic risk). Although 6–12 ECT treatments are usually sufficient for major depression, standard practice is to continue treatment until the patient responds; further treatment after this point is unnecessary and may produce intolerable cognitive impairment. An early practice of estimating the "dose" in ECT by the number of seizure seconds was not supported by later research.

ECT is usually recommended for depressed patients who have not responded to antidepressants, because the expectation is that it will be effective when medications were not. However, comparisons of patients who received adequate doses of antidepressants (or antidepressant–antipsychotic combinations for psychotic depression) with those who underwent inadequate medication trials demonstrated that about 90% of the latter responded to ECT, whereas the response rate was only about 50% for patients who received adequate antidepressant doses (Devanand et al. 1991). The assumption that patients who were unresponsive to a particular antidepressant before ECT respond to that medication after ECT was contradicted by the same research, which showed that antidepressants are no more effective after ECT than they were before ECT. However, a patient's ability to tolerate an antidepressant may be enhanced by ECT. Maintenance therapy involving continued ECT or adequate doses of medications that either have not been tried or were not found to be ineffective previously is necessary to prevent relapse and recurrence of depression. Maintenance ECT is safe, effective in preventing relapse and recurrence, and especially useful in elderly patients, who tolerate maintenance pharmacotherapy poorly.

The most common side effects of ECT, confusion and memory loss, are more pronounced after bilateral ECT. Anterograde amnesia is most obvious within 45 minutes of a treatment, but loss of memory of events occurring from a few days to as long as 2 years before ECT (i.e., retrograde amnesia) also occurs. In some cases, personally significant memories from the recent or even the distant past (i.e., autobiographical memory) may be lost permanently. Most of the time, however, cognitive functioning after recovery from the acute effects of ECT is better than it was before treatment, as a result of recovery from the cognitive impairment of depression. A small group of patients complain of severe cognitive disruption that cannot be demonstrated on objective testing. Because these patients also have not had remission of depression, their cognitive symptoms may represent residual depressive symptoms or perhaps awareness of subtle deficits that nondepressed individuals would ignore. There is no evidence from studies of cerebral structure or function that ECT as it is currently administered causes brain damage (Coffey et al. 1991).

Repetitive Transcranial Magnetic Stimulation

The hypothesis that the pathophysiology of depression involves in part hypoactivity of the left prefrontal cortex led to the application of a potent local magnetic field, which induces a localized electrical current perpendicular to the magnetic field, over that region (Mosimann et al. 2000). Preliminary studies of motor evoked potential threshold suggest that changes in brain activity may occur at sites remote from the stimulus without a generalized electrical seizure in the brain. Animal studies demonstrate upregulation of β-adrenergic receptors in the frontal cortex and downregulation of the same receptors in the striatum and downregulation of 5-HT$_2$ receptors in the frontal cortex (Ben-Shachar et al. 1999). The fact that these receptor effects differ from those of other antidepressant treatments may indicate that rTMS has a different mechanism of action or that receptor actions are not the primary mediators of antidepressant action. High-frequency (20 Hz) rTMS, which increases brain glucose metabolism and regional blood flow, has been found to be more effective in the treatment of major depression than low-frequency (1 Hz) rTMS.

In open studies, rTMS significantly improved depressive symptoms in patients with refractory depression but had no effect on mood in healthy subjects (Mosimann et al. 2000). A random assignment crossover comparison of active and sham high-frequency rTMS found that the active treatment reduced Hamilton Rating Scale for Depression (Ham-D) scores by five points, compared with a three-point reduction during sham treatment (George et al. 1997). On the other hand, when real and sham rTMS were compared in a 2-week double-blind study (4 weeks of real rTMS followed), a lack of difference was noted between the groups because of a high rate of spontaneous improvement in all subjects (Loo et al. 1999). rTMS is theoretically appealing because it does not have cognitive side effects (the only important adverse effects are headache and, rarely, seizures), but most studies are of very short duration and involve small numbers of subjects, limiting interpretation of the data.

Artificial Bright Light

Artificial bright light is an effective treatment for seasonal affective disorder (SAD), for which remission rates in published studies range from 36% to 75% (Rosenthal and Oren 1995). The minimal intensity of light that appears necessary for an antidepressant effect is 2,500 lux (1 lux = 1 lumen per square meter) placed about 1 m from the patient. At greater intensities of light, a shorter duration of exposure to the light appears necessary. For example, remission rates with 30 minutes of a 10,000-lux light are similar to those with 2,500 lux for 2 hours (Tam et al. 1995). To be effective, light must enter the patient's eyes. Although the hypothesis that light acts through retinohypothalamic pathways to normalize a phase delay in melatonin secretion has been questioned, phase advancing of the sleep–wake cycle with morning bright light probably is a mechanism of action in some cases (Rosenthal and Oren 1995). A light visor is available that has a lower intensity of light but is closer to the eyes than the standard light box, but the 35%–40% rate of response to light-visor treatment is no better than the response rate achieved with placebo. Use of an "artificial dawn," in which light of gradually increasing intensity is turned on before the patient wakes up, may be useful but is not as effective as standard light therapy.

Some patients respond exclusively to morning light, and some respond equally well to light administered at any time of the day, but few patients respond preferentially to evening light. Some authorities recommend that the patient start treatment at whatever time of day is most convenient, so that compliance is increased, whereas others think that morning light should be tried first, especially in the case of patients who tend to sleep late. Exposure to light too late in the day may make it difficult to fall asleep. There do not appear to be clinically significant differences in the effectiveness of any particular wavelength of light or of full-spectrum light versus cool-white fluorescent light.

Many patients respond to bright light within 3–5 days and relapse if they discontinue the light treatment for 3 days in a row during the winter. However, some patients who do not respond after 1 week of treatment respond during the second week (Labbate et al. 1995). Patients with bipolar SAD may have better responses to artificial bright light than patients with unipolar SAD. Nonseasonally depressed patients may not respond to light therapy as well as patients with SAD, but chronically depressed patients with fall-winter exacerbations of depression may benefit from this treatment, at least as an adjunct. Artificial bright light may also be useful for treating seasonal lethargy without obvious depression, midwinter insomnia, jet lag, adaptation to work shift changes, and abnormal sleep–wake cycles in bipolar disorder.

Artificial bright light appears to be safe if it does not contain light in the ultraviolet spectrum. The most common side effects are headache and nausea; fatigue due to alteration of the sleep–wake cycle may occur acutely but often remits after about a week. Concerns that lithium might make the retina more subject to damage from artificial bright light have not been borne out by recent research. Like anything with antidepressant properties, artificial bright light has the potential to induce mania or hypomania in patients with bipolar disorder (Rosenthal and Oren 1995).

Novel Treatments

Augmentation of antidepressants with 25–50 µg of triiodothyronine (T_3) has been said to improve refractory depression in as many as two-thirds of cases (Prange 1996). Although most patients who have been reported to respond to T_3 augmentation have been grossly euthyroid, it is not known how many might have had subclinical forms of hypothyroidism as indicated by thyroid-stimulating hormone levels or results of a thyrotropin-releasing hormone stimulation test (Prange 1996).

Because of the importance of the membrane inositol phosphate system in intracellular signaling involving G proteins and calcium ions, observations that lithium reduces inositol biphosphate turnover by inhibiting inositol-1-phosphatase, and reports of reduced cerebrospinal fluid inositol levels in depression, a number of small trials of inositol in mood disorders have been conducted. In a 4-week study involving 28 patients randomly assigned to inositol 12 g/day or placebo, improvement of Ham-D scores was significantly greater in the inositol treatment group (Levine et al. 1995). By contrast, in another trial involving 22 patients with bipolar depression, the likelihood of a 50% reduction in Ham-D scores was greater among patients treated with high doses of inositol than among patients receiving placebo, but the differences were not statistically significant (Chengappa et al. 2000). In a double-blind trial, depressed patients who did not respond to SSRIs alone also did not improve when inositol was added (Nemets et al. 1999). On the basis of a hypothesis of imbalance between phosphatidylinositol and phosphatidylcholine second messengers, 6 patients with rapid cycling who were being treated with choline bitartrate were given lithium as well. In the 4 patients who exhibited reduction of affective symptoms, the concentration of choline-containing compounds increased in the basal ganglia as measured by magnetic resonance spectroscopy. In an open study of 11 patients with refractory mania, hypomania, or mixed states, addition of donepezil, a cholinesterase inhibitor, to mood stabilizers led to marked improvement in 6 or slight improvement in 3 (Burt et al. 1999).

In eight randomized controlled trials, St. John's wort *(Hypericum)* was more effective than placebo but less effective than TCAs in treating major depression of mild to moderate severity (Gaster and Holroyd 2000). In a 6-week British study, 324 outpatients with mild major depression were randomly assigned to imipramine 150 mg/day or 500 mg of a standardized preparation of *Hypericum* extract per day (Woelk 2000). Mean Ham-D scores decreased by about 50% in both groups, but St. John's wort was better tolerated and was more effective in reducing anxiety. The absence of a placebo group, the lack of a complete response in either group, and the relatively mild nature of the depression limited interpretation of the data. One of these deficiencies was corrected in an 8-week American multicenter study involving outpatients with major depression of slightly higher severity who were randomly assigned to placebo or 1,200 mg of standardized *Hypericum* extract per day (Shelton et al. 2001a). Reductions in rating scale scores for depression and anxiety did not differ between the groups. Although St. John's wort is usually well tolerated, it may interact with highly serotonergic antidepressants and MAOIs, and occasional cases of apparent serotonin syndrome have been reported.

Observations of increased activity of the hypothalamic-pituitary-adrenal axis in major depression suggest that medications that inhibit cortisol production or action could improve depression. In 28 reports of antiglucocorticoid treatment of Cushing's syndrome, improvement of depression was noted in as many as 70% of patients (Wolkowitz and Reus 1999). A combination of aminoglutethimide, metyrapone, and/or ketoconazole, all of which interfere with cortisol synthesis, when administered along with maintenance exogenous cortisol improved severe refractory major depression in 11 of 17 patients in one open trial (Murphy 1997). A few small open trials of corticotropin-releasing factor inhibitors in refractory depression at least support the possibility that such approaches may reduce some depressive symptoms (Wolkowitz and Reus 1999), although this kind of treatment obviously is not without substantial risks. Open clinical experience suggests that mifepristone (RU-486), a glucocorticoid receptor antagonist, produced rapid relief of refractory depression in a small number of patients (Murphy et al. 1995). This substance, which was recently released in the United States as an emergency contraceptive and abortifacient, produces its gynecological effect by blocking progesterone receptors, but it also antagonizes cortisol receptors.

S-Adenosylmethionine (SAMe) is a product of methionine metabolism that participates in transmethylation, transsulfuration, and transaminophosphorylation. Reports of reduced cerebrospinal fluid levels of SAMe in depressed patients led to a series of clinical trials of supplemental SAMe for depression. Double-blind comparisons of parenteral SAMe with placebo and several TCAs suggested efficacy in major depression. When high doses of oral SAMe were compared with imipramine therapy and desipramine therapy in depressed patients, similar degrees of improvement were noted (Bell et al. 1994), but in the absence of a placebo group it is difficult to know whether this might have occurred with high doses of any substance. Observations of mania induced by SAMe support a possible antidepressant action of this substance. Although there are insufficient data to support the use of SAMe as a first-line agent for depression, it may be worth considering for patients who do not do well with standard antidepressants.

Recent studies have suggested that there are decreased concentrations of omega-3 fatty acids and decreased ratios of omega-3 to omega-6 fatty acids in the plasma and erythrocytes of patients with major depression (Peet et al. 1998). In some of these studies, severity of depression has been negatively correlated with both red blood cell membrane levels and dietary intake of n-3 polyunsaturated fatty acids. One hypothesis is that alterations of unsaturated fatty acids in depression are related to a nonspecific inflammatory response that has been associated with decreased availability of serum tryptophan. Although alterations of membrane fatty acids could alter membrane fluidity and therefore intracellular signaling, adequate treatment of depression does not seem to alter fatty acid composition. No placebo-controlled studies have yet shown that treatment with omega-3 fatty acids improves depression.

Pramipexole, a dopaminergic agent used to treat Parkinson's disease, has been used by some clinicians as an antidepressant. Fifty percent of 12 depressed patients with bipolar disorder and 40% of 20 patients with unipolar depression whose charts were studied in a retrospective review had antidepressant responses to this medication, administered for 24 weeks at a mean dose of 0.7 mg/day (Sporn et al. 2000).

Effects of substance P antagonists on dorsal raphe serotonergic neurons similar to the effects observed with antidepressants have led to trials of a number of antagonists of the neurokinin-1 (NK1) substance P receptor as possible antidepressants (Haddjeri and Blier 2001). MK-869 was the first of these to be shown to be effective for major depressive disorder (Rupniak 2002). This compound, which was found in one study to be as effective as a comparison SSRI (Lieb et al. 2000), may also have anxiolytic properties. If current Phase III placebo-controlled studies support an antidepressant effect of NK1 antagonists, the role of these medications in fibromyalgia and other depressive symptoms associated with chronic pain will be of particular interest.

■ TREATMENTS FOR BIPOLAR DISORDER

Medications

Medications that are used to treat mania (i.e., antimanic drugs) are also used to prevent or reduce the frequency of affective recurrences in bipolar disorder, in which case they are called *mood stabilizers.* Although truly long-term data from well-designed randomized clinical trials are not available for mood-stabilizing actions of antimanic drugs other than lithium, a consensus panel of 58 national experts strongly agreed that antimanic drugs should be used in all phases of treatment of bipolar disorder, including depression (Sachs et al. 2000). An antimanic action of a medication, which may result from sedative and antipsychotic effects rather than a primary action on the mood disorder, does not necessarily predict subsequent mood stabilization, which implies an antirecurrence action. Studies of new antimanic and mood-stabilizing medications may not be comparable to older studies because some newer studies include more patients with refractory mood disorders, whereas industry-sponsored projects attempt to exclude patients with refractory illnesses.

Lithium

Lithium, the best studied of the antimanic drugs, has well-established efficacy as an antimanic drug and as a prophylactic agent against recurrences of mania and bipolar depression. Lithium may reduce depressive recurrences in highly recurrent unipolar depression, and it reduces the risk of suicide among patients with mood disorders. Lithium appears to be most effective in patients with complete remissions between episodes and without mixed mania, rapid cycling, and a need for antipsychotics. Even when it is effective, more than 50% of lithium-treated patients have another affective episode within 2 years, and the prophylactic effect of the drug is attenuated over time in 20%–40% of patients (Goldberg et al. 1996). Discontinuation of lithium (and probably other mood stabilizers), especially if it is rapid, can result in rebound of the mood disorder as well as refractoriness to the therapeutic effect of the medication in some (Hopkins and Gelenberg 1994; Post 1990) but not all (Berghofer and Muller-Oerlinghausen 2000) patients.

Lithium doses are adjusted by serum level. Although some studies suggest that trough levels greater than 0.8 mEq/L are associated with greater efficacy, if more side effects (Gelenberg et al. 1989), other research suggests that levels greater than 0.8 mEq/L may not be more effective than levels of 0.5–0.8 mEq/L, possibly because of higher drop-out rates at the higher levels (Vestergaard et al. 1998). Common adverse effects of lithium at therapeutic levels include polydipsia, polyuria, hypothyroidism, hyperparathyroidism, tremor, impaired cognitive function, nausea, and weight gain. Weight gain and interference with insulin receptor signaling make lithium therapy problematic for diabetic patients, whereas cognitive dysfunction, which can occur in as many as 50% of patients who take lithium chronically, can be a significant problem for students. Lithium toxicity, which becomes more likely when serum levels exceed 1.5 mEq/L, causes coarse tremor, ataxia, vertigo, dysarthria, vomiting, delirium, muscle fasciculations, and cardiotoxicity and may be fatal. Debate continues about whether chronic lithium therapy causes nephrotoxicity, but permanent neurotoxicity after lithium intoxication has been reported (Saxena and Mallikarjuna 1988). The 24-hour elimination half-life of chronically administered lithium permits once-daily dosing, which may reduce the frequency of adverse effects.

Although the rate of response of uncomplicated mania to lithium in three trials ranged from 59% to 91%, response rates among patients with mixed states and rapid cycling were only 29%–43% (Gershon and Soares 1997). However, in a prospective study involving 360 patients and an average of 8.8 years of follow-up, even though patients with rapid cycling continued to have more affective episodes than patients without rapid cycling and the overall remission rate was less than 30%, lithium treatment was associated with similar rates of reduction of affective episodes, psychiatric hospitalization, and time ill among patients with and patients without rapid cycling, and there was no difference between the two groups in terms of lack of any response to lithium (Baldessarini et al. 2000). The authors attributed the better response to lithium by this particular sample of patients with rapid cycling to conservative use of antidepressants, high rates of compliance, and an absence of comorbid substance dependence.

Anticonvulsants

The anticonvulsants carbamazepine and valproate (divalproex) (Table 4–6) have been widely studied as antimanic drugs and mood stabilizers (Bowden 1995; Okuma et al. 1990). Alone or in combination with each other or with lithium, the anticonvulsants may be more frequently effective than lithium in mixed mania, rapid-cycling bipolar disorder, and refractory bipolar disorder. Nonspecific electroencephalographic changes, even in patients who do not have seizure disorders, predict a better response to valproate than lithium (Reeves 2001). More rapid dose escalation may be possible with valproate than with lithium and carbamazepine; this could result in faster achievement of therapeutic levels and possibly earlier discharge of hospitalized manic patients. One protocol calls for rapid oral loading with divalproex 20 mg/kg/day for the first 5 days of treatment (Keck et al. 1993). This approach leads to achievement of steady-state levels during the initial phase of treatment and more rapid symptom reduction in mania, although a significant amount of improvement of agitation, insomnia, and other manic

TABLE 4–6. **Some antimanic drugs**

Generic name	Trade name	Usual daily dose (mg)	Therapeutic level
Carbamazepine	Tegretol	600–3,000	?4–12 µg/mL
Divalproex	Depakote	750–5,000	100 µg/mL
Lithium	Lithobid, Eskalith	600–3,000	0.5–1.2 mEq/L
Nimodipine	Nimotop	180–720	—
Olanzapine	Zyprexa	10–20	—
Verapamil	Isoptin, Calan	360–480	—

symptoms may be attributable to sedation. Studies with findings supporting briefer hospitalizations of patients treated primarily with valproate versus those treated with lithium (Keck et al. 1996) have not controlled for the fact that valproate became a common treatment for mania at the same time that inpatient lengths of stay began to decrease substantially as a result of managed care, new therapeutic philosophies, and other changes in the hospital treatment of mania. Controlled trials support the antimanic action of valproate in mixed states more than that of carbamazepine, and the prophylactic effect of carbamazepine more than that of valproate (Licht 1998).

The most troublesome adverse effects of valproate are sedation and weight gain. Less common but equally troublesome side effects are cognitive impairment and hair loss. An issue that has been discussed widely concerns the relationship between valproate and polycystic ovary syndrome. In a Finnish prospective study (Isojarvi et al. 1993), 238 women undergoing treatment for epilepsy were evaluated for polycystic ovaries (by ultrasound) and hyperandrogenism, which can be associated with valproate therapy and which is a risk factor for polycystic ovary syndrome. Eighty percent of women who began taking valproate before age 20 had polycystic ovaries or hyperandrogenism. In contrast, only 27% of women treated with other anticonvulsants before age 20 had identical profiles. Of women who began treatment after age 20, a total of 56% of those receiving valproate had polycystic ovaries or hyperandrogenism, compared with 20% of those not receiving valproate. The incidence of polycystic ovaries in both samples was higher than the maximum reported rate of polycystic ovaries in women with epilepsy (40%). It is not known whether polycystic ovaries demonstrated by ultrasound in this study conveyed an increased risk of problems encountered in spontaneous polycystic ovary syndrome—namely, hirsutism, anovulation, menstrual irregularities, insulin resistance, carbohydrate intolerance, and an increased risk of endometrial cancer.

Some studies suggest that carbamazepine is more effective than lithium for rapid cycling (Kleindienst and Greil 2000). However, other research indicates that it is not superior to lithium for this indication (Okuma 1993). On the basis of clinical experience, open trials, and retrospective chart reviews, expert consensus panels now recommend initiating treatment of rapid cycling with divalproex (Bowden et al. 2001; Expert Consensus Panel for Bipolar Disorder 1996), which appears to be equally effective in rapid- and non-rapid-cycling bipolar disorder (Bowden et al. 1994).

One study suggested that the therapeutic level of valproate in the treatment of acute mania might be around 100 µg/mL, which is achieved with daily doses of 750–5,000 mg (Bowden et al. 1994). The frequently reported therapeutic level of 50–125 µg/mL is actually a normal level (i.e., the usual range found when levels are tested) and has not been shown to be correlated with clinical response in epilepsy or bipolar disorder. An elimination half-life of less than a day often necessitates twice-daily dosing, although a significant number of patients respond to a single bedtime dose, possibly because of a dynamic half-life that is longer than the elimination half-life. An extended-release form of divalproex (Depakote ER) was recently made available. With once-daily dosing, it has been shown to be as effective as immediate-release divalproex in the treatment of epilepsy, but it has not been formally investigated in mood disorders. This preparation may be associated with a lower incidence of weight gain than the immediate-release form, but because the smallest dose is 500 mg, initiating therapy gradually still involves use of the immediate-release preparation.

The dose of carbamazepine (usually 400–1,200 mg/day) is frequently adjusted on the basis of serum level, but there is no scientific evidence of a specific therapeutic level for carbamazepine in epilepsy, let alone mood disorders. On the other hand, higher serum levels are associated with more psychomotor impairment. Obtaining periodic complete blood counts and then withdrawing carbamazepine if the white blood cell count decreases to less than 3,000 cells/mm^3 will not prevent agranulocytosis, because this extremely rare (1 in 100,000 to 1 in 250,000) event occurs abruptly and is not correlated with the benign, gradual, and transient decrease in white blood cells that takes place during the first few months of carbamazepine treatment in about 20% of patients. During treatment with anticonvulsants, routine performance of liver function tests is not cost-effective because hepatotoxicity is rarely caused by these drugs, and when it is, it can be better identified by clinical observation than by laboratory testing (Hoshino et al. 1995). Use of anticonvulsants during pregnancy is associated with a 7%–10% risk of fetal neural tube defects, cardiac anomalies, and cognitive deficits (Lindhout and Omtzigt 1992). Folic acid supplementation may reduce these risks but does not make anticonvulsants safe during pregnancy.

Lamotrigine and gabapentin, two new anticonvulsants that have been approved in the United States as adjuncts in the treatment of refractory epilepsy, have been used recently in clinical settings to treat bipolar illness. Positive effects of lamotrigine and gabapentin on mood are suggested by reports that patients in continuation studies elect more often to keep taking these medications than would be expected on the basis of improved seizure control alone, apparently because of an improved sense of well-being.

In a few cases and open series described in the literature, gabapentin was associated with improvement of mood in bipolar disorder (Altshuler et al. 1999). However, controlled studies have not confirmed this impression. In a crossover comparison of lamotrigine, gabapentin, and placebo, administered for 6 weeks to patients with refractory mood disorders, significantly more patients (52%) improved with lamotrigine than with gabapentin (26%), the latter drug being equivalent in efficacy to placebo (23%) (Frye et al.

2000). A placebo-controlled trial of gabapentin added to lithium, valproate, or a combination of the two in bipolar I disorder found that gabapentin was no better than placebo in reducing mania, hypomania, mixed states, or depression (Pande et al. 2000). Clinical experience suggests that gabapentin is more effective as an antidepressant and an anxiolytic than as a mood stabilizer, although it may be a useful adjunct for some patients with chronic bipolar illness and predominant depression.

Potential mechanisms of a positive effect of lamotrigine in bipolar disorder include inhibition of glutamate release and calcium-channel blockade. Lamotrigine was found in controlled trials to be more effective than placebo in bipolar depression (Calabrese et al. 1999b), and a small controlled study suggested efficacy in mania (Berk 1999). In a 48-week open trial of lamotrigine therapy as adjunctive treatment ($n=60$) or monotherapy ($n=15$) in patients with bipolar I and bipolar II disorder, depressed patients had a mean reduction in depression scores of 42%, and patients with hypomania, mania, or mixed states had on average a 74% reduction in mania rating scores (Calabrese et al. 1999a). A group treated with a comparison medication and a placebo group would be necessary to be confident in the long-term efficacy of lamotrigine.

Open observation of seven patients with rapid cycling treated with lithium and seven treated with lamotrigine revealed that although 43% of lithium-treated patients had fewer than four affective episodes over the following year, 86% of lamotrigine-treated patients had fewer than four episodes (Walden et al. 2000). However, the small number of subjects and the open method limit interpretation of these findings. In a recent complicated trial, patients with rapid cycling were stabilized with a variety of treatments and then were randomly assigned to monotherapy with lamotrigine or placebo in a double-blind protocol (Calabrese et al. 2000). A total of 41% of lamotrigine-treated patients, versus 26% of patients who received placebo, remained relapse free for 6 months of prospective treatment.

In a multicenter open trial of lamotrigine monotherapy that was supported by the manufacturer, 200–500 mg of lamotrigine was added to or substituted for ongoing medications for 48 weeks in 75 patients with bipolar disorder who were unresponsive to or intolerant of the pharmacotherapy they were receiving (Bowden et al. 1999). During the preceding 12 months, 55% of these patients had met DSM-IV (American Psychiatric Association 1994) criteria for rapid cycling. Compared with the 6% of patients without rapid cycling dropped out of the study because of lack of efficacy, 22% of rapid-cycling patients dropped out for this reason and 71% of lamotrigine-treated patients versus 38% of the other patients did not complete the study for any reason. Lamotrigine was associated with better improvement of depressive than manic symptoms, and severe manic symptoms showed little response. The overall rate (58%) of at least some improvement with lamotrigine among rapid-cycling patients was probably attributable to the fact that patients with rapid cycling were more than twice as likely as other patients to have persistent depression than persistent mania or hypomania. The finding that depression seems to improve more than mania in these studies suggests that lamotrigine may be more useful for patients with rapid cycling who are predominantly depressed, a possibility that finds support in the observation that lithium was superior to placebo in preventing recurrences of mania over 18 months, whereas lamotrigine was superior to placebo in reducing recurrences of depression (Bowden et al. 2001).

The most frequent adverse effects of lamotrigine and gabapentin include dizziness, headache, diplopia, ataxia, nausea, amblyopia, somnolence, fatigue, ataxia, rash, weight gain, and vomiting. The manufacturer raised concerns about dangerous allergic rashes with the use of lamotrigine, a risk that is substantially reduced by slower dosage escalation (12.5 mg/week) than was originally recommended. A primary antidepressant action of gabapentin is supported by reports that it has induced mania (Leweke et al. 1999) and was associated with aggressive behavior, hyperactivity, and tantrums in a number of children, most of whom had a diagnosis of attention-deficit/hyperactivity disorder (Lee et al. 1996).

Expert opinion has favored adjunctive use of other anticonvulsants such as topiramate in the treatment of rapid cycling. The only data in favor of this application come from a few case reports and case series (McElroy et al. 2000), and there is no controlled evidence that it is effective for this indication. Topiramate can be useful as an appetite suppressant for some patients who gain weight with other medications. However, it may contribute to mood destabilization in some patients, and cognitive impairment can be a limiting side effect. Oxcarbazepine, an analogue of carbamazepine that appears to have fewer adverse effects and interactions while being as effective as an anticonvulsant, has increasingly been used as a mood stabilizer. Only two prospective 2-week trials of oxcarbazepine in mania have been reported on in the literature (reviewed in Dietrich et al. 2001), one finding that oxcarbazepine 1,400 mg/day was equivalent to lithium 1,100 mg/day, and the other that oxcarbazepine 2,100 mg/day was equivalent to haloperidol 42 mg/day. Although oxcarbazepine has not yet been reported to cause bone marrow suppression, a risk of hyponatremia warrants caution in patients with compulsive water drinking.

Calcium Channel–Blocking Agents

Observations of hyperactive intracellular calcium signaling in bipolar disorder and calcium antagonist properties of mood stabilizers such as lithium and carbamazepine led to studies of calcium-channel antagonists in bipolar disorder. Reports of double-blind trials of verapamil in manic or hypomanic individuals have been published (Dubovsky et al. 1986). In two 4- to 5-week double-blind trials, verapamil and lithium were found to have equivalent antimanic efficacy. Verapamil and nimodipine have been noted to have mood-stabilizing properties in some manic and rapid-cycling patients (Barton and Gitlin 1987; Manna 1991). Experience with verapamil suggests that it is most effective in patients who have responded to lithium; patients with refractory mood disorders usually respond poorly to this drug as a single agent. In one trial, verapamil appeared to be less effective than lithium in the treatment of acute mania, but the results were limited by small absolute numerical differences between groups in rating scale scores, P values that would not usually be considered significant with the statistical measures used in the study, and the absence of any differences between mania rating-scale scores in the lithium and verapamil treatment groups. The finding of a double-blind study that verapamil was not superior to placebo (Janicak et al. 1998) could reflect either a lack of efficacy in this population or the inclusion of patients with lithium therapy–refractory illness, who usually do not respond to verapamil. Conversely, an open-label study of verapamil in 28 women who refused treatment with lithium and anticonvulsants found that verapamil significantly reduced treated manic or hypomanic symptoms in pure mania/hypomania and in mixed states but was ineffective for depression (Wisner et al. 2002).

The dose range of verapamil that has most frequently been found to be effective in bipolar mood disorders is 360–480 mg/day. A short elimination half-life necessitates dosing four times daily; the sustained-release formulation of verapamil is not predictably effective for mood disorders. The most common side effects are related to vasodilation and include dizziness, headache, skin flushing, tachycardia, and nausea. In randomized trials of calcium-channel blockers for maternal hypertension, premature labor, and fetal arrhythmias during pregnancy, no evidence of teratogenesis was found, nor were there significant effects on uterine or placental blood flow. In two published reports of the use of verapamil in pregnant patients, good control of mania in three manic women and uneventful delivery of healthy infants occurred after sustained-release verapamil was administered during pregnancy (Goodnick 1993; Wisner et al. 2002).

Nimodipine, a highly lipophilic dihydropyridine calcium-channel blocker, has been studied in a few small trials involving patients with unstable bipolar disorder. It has been speculated that a mild anticonvulsant effect may contribute to the benefit of this medication, but this hypothesis has not been confirmed. As described in the single case report in the literature, an adolescent boy with ultradian (ultrarapid) cycling had "marked" improvement of mood swings while taking nimodipine 180 mg/day with adjunctive thyroxine (T_4), and this improvement persisted over 36 months of follow-up (Davanzo et al. 1999). In an open prospective study, 12 patients with rapid cycling took part in three 6-month trials: a trial of lithium alone, one of nimodipine alone, and a trial of both medications (Manna 1991). Although all three medications reduced affective recurrences compared with baseline, the combination was significantly more effective than either drug alone.

In a study involving 13 patients with refractory mood disorders, 3 of whom had ultradian cycling and 5 of whom had continuous rapid cycling (a distinction that may not be clinically important), nimodipine at doses up to 720 mg/day was completely or partially effective in reducing recurrences of mania and depression in all patients with ultradian or continuous cycling but in only 1 of 5 patients with more classic rapid cycling, and blind substitution of placebo resulted in relapse; nimodipine was also completely effective in reducing recurrences in subjects with recurrent brief depression (Pazzaglia et al. 1993). In an extension of this study, 10 of 30 patients with refractory mood disorders (mostly bipolar) had "moderate to marked" responses to nimodipine administered blindly, but not to placebo (Pazzaglia et al. 1993). Of 14 patients who did not respond to nimodipine monotherapy (11 of whom had rapid-cycling bipolar mood disorders), 29% had more robust responses when carbamazepine was added to nimodipine. The combination of carbamazepine and nimodipine seemed most effective in patients with rapid or ultradian cycling, unipolar recurrent brief depression, or bipolar depression (one case). Blind substitution for nimodipine of verapamil (which acts on different calcium-channel blocker receptors) led to relapse, but substitutions of isradipine, which acts on the same receptor, was associated with maintenance of remission.

Because it has an elimination half-life of 3 hours, nimodipine should be administered frequently to maintain a steady-state concentration. Clinical experience suggests that nimodipine may be particularly useful in combination with other mood stabilizers in the treatment of patients with ultradian cycling. This medication is generally well tolerated, the most common side effects being vasomotor symptoms such as flushing of the skin. At more than $5.50 per pill, nimodipine is prohibitively expensive. However, the patent has expired, and a somewhat cheaper generic preparation is available.

Antipsychotic Drugs

Case reports, studies, and reviews have suggested that chlorproma-
zine, haloperidol, pimozide, thiothixene, and thioridazine have applications alone or as adjuncts to lithium in acute treatment of
mania (McElroy et al. 1996). After conducting a critical review,
Licht (1998) concluded that randomized controlled trials demonstrate that all neuroleptics have antimanic properties, especially as
adjuncts; however, the efficacy of neuroleptic therapy as maintenance treatment is not well demonstrated in controlled studies. Naturalistic follow-up studies found that 34%–95% of patients continue
to take neuroleptics alone or in combination with lithium 6–12 months
after an index manic episode (Sernyak and Woods 1993). Although
some experts infer that the frequent use of neuroleptics in bipolar
disorder indicates that improper use of these medications is common, it is also possible that many patients need neuroleptic drugs
for prevention of affective recurrence even if psychosis has remitted, as is true of psychotic unipolar depression, or that the lack of
other effective therapies for many patients leads to frequent use
of neuroleptics as a last resort.

Common problems that occur when patients with bipolar disorder are treated with neuroleptics include increased risks of tardive
dyskinesia and neuroleptic malignant syndrome, as well as neurotoxic interactions with lithium. In addition, concern has been raised
that chronic neuroleptic use could be associated with withdrawal or
supersensitivity (tardive) psychoses that are presumably caused by
supersensitivity of postsynaptic dopamine receptors. Most putative
cases of tardive psychoses have been reported in schizophrenic patients in whom chronic neuroleptic use was thought to induce rather
than prevent psychotic relapses (Miller and Chouinard 1993).
Whereas tardive psychosis is rare, if it occurs at all, more concern
has been raised that continuing neuroleptic therapy for too long
could make manic patients prone to more severe and prolonged depressive episodes and rapid cycling (McElroy et al. 1996).

Clozapine, an atypical antipsychotic drug with complex actions, appears to have antimanic and mood-stabilizing effects in

nonpsychotic as well as psychotic patients with bipolar or schizoaffective disorders. Response rates average around 69% (Ghaemi and Goodwin 1999). Clozapine has been found useful for treating non-rapid-cycling, rapid-cycling, and refractory bipolar disorder (Green et al. 2000). In a random-assignment, open, year-long comparison of the addition of clozapine to "usual treatment" versus usual treatment alone in refractory bipolar disorder with or without psychosis, clozapine improved affective symptoms significantly (Suppes et al. 1999). There is insufficient experience to confirm observations that clozapine therapy is better prophylaxis against recurrent mania than against recurrent depression, but this observation has been made about most mood-stabilizing treatments. In contrast, clozapine has not been reported to induce mania or rapid cycling.

Adverse effects of clozapine, the need for frequent laboratory monitoring, and the potential for enhancement of a crowded market for antipsychotic drugs have stimulated interest in the newer atypical antipsychotic agents as possible adjunctive mood stabilizers. In four studies, an average of 51% of patients with bipolar disorder responded to adjunctive treatment with risperidone (Ghaemi and Goodwin 1999). Such positive results have involved low doses and trials that were probably too brief for any antidepressant properties of risperidone to predominate over the drug's sedating and antipsychotic effects. The finding of an apparent antimanic effect of olanzapine in two industry-sponsored double-blind comparisons with placebo (Tohen et al. 1999, 2000), supplemented by findings of a 4-week randomized comparison of olanzapine and lithium (Berk et al. 1999), along with the overall weighted average response rates of 50% in the three controlled studies just mentioned (Ghaemi and Goodwin 1999), has led to claims that these atypical antipsychotic drugs are mood stabilizers. This impression was strengthened by a 3-week, randomized, double-blind comparison of olanzapine and divalproex in hospitalized patients with mania or mixed states (Tohen et al. 2002). Patients treated with olanzapine had significantly greater mean improvement of mania rating scale scores and significantly olanzapine-treated patients had remission (defined as a level of symptomatology equivalent to hypomania). However, only 54% of olanzapine-treated patients (compared with 42% of divalproex-treated patients) had at least a 50% reduction in manic symptoms. Open adjunctive treatment with an average of 8 mg/day of olanzapine added to mood stabilizers resulted in significant reductions in manic and depressive symptoms over 43 weeks of follow-up (Vieta et al. 2001), but the absence of a comparison group makes it difficult to know how important the olanzapine was to the outcome, and there is as yet no evidence that monotherapy with this medication is effective for mood stabilization.

Because other antipsychotic medications, benzodiazepines, and clonidine have all been found to be effective for acute mania, it seems unlikely that a putative antimanic action of atypical antipsychotics is specific to these medications. One issue that requires further study is the possibility that even if sedative and antipsychotic properties may be helpful for mania, antidepressant properties demonstrated in multicenter schizophrenia trials of most atypical antipsychotics could eventually overcome any potential antimanic effect and lead to mood destabilization. This concern is supported to some extent by a number of reports of mania apparently induced by risperidone and olanzapine (Dwight et al. 1994; Simon et al. 1999). Although most clinicians prefer to try the easier-to-use, newer atypical antipsychotic drugs first, clozapine appears to be more consistently effective than the newer antipsychotic drugs for stabilizing mood in patients with more severe refractory forms of bipolar mood disorder. If other atypical antipsychotic medications are used chronically, lower doses may be less likely to destabilize mood.

Benzodiazepines

In the treatment of acute mania, addition of benzodiazepines, especially lorazepam and clonazepam, to antipsychotic drugs appears to provide more rapid control of agitation than antipsychotics alone. Addition of benzodiazepines reduces the antipsychotic requirement but does not necessarily result in fewer extrapyramidal side effects, and benzodiazepines can have neurotoxic interactions with lithium.

Benzodiazepines have not been shown to have benefits other than improvement of sleep, agitation, and anxiety in patients with bipolar mood disorder. Tolerance may develop to the psychotropic as well as the antiepileptic effects of clonazepam. Although most benzodiazepines are probably equally useful in bipolar disorder, alprazolam may have antidepressant properties that can lead to mania and possibly increased cycling in some patients. With the increasing use of atypical antipsychotic drugs that are better tolerated at higher doses than neuroleptics in the treatment of mania, benzodiazepines have been prescribed less frequently for acute mania and are mainly used as sleeping pills or anxiolytics in the long-term treatment of bipolar disorder.

These uses of benzodiazepines can be more complex than might be apparent. Treating insomnia can contribute to mood stability, but clonazepam, which is frequently used as a hypnotic in bipolar disorder, can aggravate depression. Failure to recognize that anxiety is a symptom of mixed hypomania in bipolar disorder rather than a separate disorder may result in a focus on anxiety relief without adequate attention to further mood stabilization.

Thyroid Hormone

The association between hypothyroidism and rapid cycling (see Chapter 2) makes it important to correct subclinical hypothyroidism in all patients with rapid cycling. Observations dating back to the 1930s (Gjessing 1938) of a positive effect of high doses of thyroid hormone on cyclical mood disorders have led some investigators to use supraphysiological doses of thyroid hormone as adjunctive treatment in rapid cycling. Open treatment with 300–500 µg of T_4 per day or 240–400 µg of T_3 per day in 10 patients with rapid cycling refractory to lithium therapy, ECT, and antipsychotic therapy led to sustained remission over 1½ to 9 years in 5 women, unsustained responses in 2 women, and no improvement in 2 men (Stancer and Persad 1982), whereas open adjunctive treatment with similar doses of L-thyroxine reduced or totally eliminated affective recurrences in patients with bipolar mood disorders (Bernstein

1992). In an open trial involving 6 patients with classic rapid cycling, the addition of levothyroxine to mood stabilizers resulted in response or remission in 4 patients that was sustained over 2 years of follow-up (Afflelou et al. 1997).

In another open protocol, 11 patients with intractable rapid cycling were treated with 150–400 μg of T_4 per day in addition to lithium, lithium and carbamazepine, antidepressants alone, a benzodiazepine alone, or antipsychotics as needed combined with other medications (Bauer and Whybrow 1990). At the beginning of the study, only 3 patients had normal thyroid function, as demonstrated in part by a thyrotropin-releasing hormone stimulation test. In all patients, adding T_4 (or increasing the existing T_4 dose, in the case of patients already taking T_4) resulted in increases in serum T_4 concentrations and decreases in thyroid-stimulating hormone concentrations into the hyperthyroid range; mania improved in 10 patients, and depression improved in 5. Of 4 patients who were then randomized to blind substitution of placebo for T_4, relapse occurred in 3.

Most patients in trials of thyroid hormone supplementation have had laboratory evidence of hypothyroidism (usually in the form of an increased thyroid-stimulating hormone level), whereas in some cases, results of thyroid tests, including a thyrotropin-releasing hormone stimulation test, were normal. To the extent that high doses of T_4 did in fact enhance the therapeutic effect of the thymoleptics, it is not clear whether this involved a primary action of the hormone or correction of central hypothyroidism in patients with poor delivery of thyroid hormone to the brain. There is no reason to think that T_4 by itself has antimanic or mood-stabilizing properties in euthyroid patients. Because excessive thyroid replacement can cause anxiety, atrial fibrillation, and osteopenia, supraphysiological doses of thyroid are usually reserved for highly refractory cases.

Electroconvulsive Therapy

Mania is the third most common indication for ECT, which is the most rapidly effective treatment for mania and the most effective treatment for bipolar depression. In a review of the published literature on the efficacy of ECT for acute mania, Mukherjee et al. (1994) found that the overall rate of "remission or marked clinical improvement" was 80% (470 of 589 patients). Interpretation of these composite figures is limited by differences in methodology and outcome measures in the studies reviewed and by the second-hand assessment of data using a nonstandard method. Although not effective for unipolar depression, lower stimulus intensities are often effective for mania.

Whereas some naturalistic studies have found that unilateral ECT was as effective as bilateral ECT for bipolar disorder (Black et al. 1987), others found bilateral ECT to be more frequently and more rapidly effective (Small et al. 1996). One reason for this discrepancy may be that shunting of current through the scalp using the Lancaster right unilateral electrode placement, which was used in at least one study showing superiority of bilateral ECT, made bilateral ECT appear less effective than if a different placement had been used. In a prospective study (Schnur et al. 1992), five of eight manic patients achieved complete remission with the d'Elia right unilateral electrode placement, which features a greater interelectrode distance, but the number of patients is too small for definitive conclusions to be drawn. However, other observations support the efficacy of right unilateral ECT in bipolar disorder. In the absence of direct comparisons between the two placements, it seems reasonable to begin with unilateral ECT, switching to bilateral ECT if right unilateral ECT does not demonstrate any benefit within a few treatments.

Once ECT with either placement has produced a remission of an acute bipolar episode, a decision about maintenance treatment must be made. Although the efficacy of mood-stabilizing medications that were not effective before ECT has not been studied in bipolar disorder as it has in unipolar depression, there is no reason to think that response to medication after ECT would be any different in the former than in the latter. Because maintenance ECT was found to be as effective as lithium in preventing manic relapse and recurrence in a prospective study and some case series (Swoboda et al. 2001), maintenance ECT seems preferable to maintenance treatment with medications in patients who did not respond to those medications before receiving ECT.

Less research has been devoted to the use of ECT in mixed states and rapid-cycling bipolar disorder. In a few cases, ECT induced remission after the patient failed to respond to thymoleptic medication. In open trials of ECT in 20 patients with mixed affective disorders resistant to lithium and/or carbamazepine therapy, ECT produced remission lasting at least 5 months in only 3 of 8 patients with rapid cycling (Mosolov and Moshchevitin 1990). An open trial of ECT in 6 patients with continuous cycling suggested that affective recurrences were more likely to be reduced when cycling began within a few months of institution of ECT than when ECT was started later in the course of rapid cycling (Wolpert et al. 1999). Although there are obvious methodological limitations, such results are consistent with clinical experience suggesting that ECT is not as effective in rapid cycling as in less complex forms of bipolar disorder, especially when the illness has been refractory to other treatments. Patients who do respond may need more ECT treatments than patients with illnesses that have not been resistant to drug therapy. Because many patients with rapid cycling are taking multiple medications, there is a greater potential for interactions with ECT.

Repetitive Transcranial Magnetic Stimulation

Data on the potential efficacy of rTMS in bipolar disorder are very sparse, although the treatment shows some promise. In 16 manic patients, fast right prefrontal rTMS resulted in significantly more improvement than fast left prefrontal rTMS, a finding that is the opposite of what has been noted in unipolar depression (Grisaru et al. 1998). Given the current lack of other studies of rTMS in bipolar disorder, this technique should be considered experimental.

Novel Treatments

Because omega-3 fatty acids, like lithium, reduce hyperactive turnover of membrane phospholipids, a possible advantage of these substances in bipolar disorder has been investigated. In the only published double-blind study, patients who received slightly less than 10 g of omega-3 fatty acids per day in addition to their standard treatment had significantly longer periods of remission than did control subjects who received placebo (Stoll et al. 1999). Many patients prefer taking fish oil in one form or another because they can prescribe this treatment for themselves, but without more data, the use of omega-3 fatty acids as adjunctive mood stabilizers must be considered experimental.

Tamoxifen, an estrogen receptor antagonist in some tissues and agonist in others, is used to prevent breast cancer recurrence and is also an inhibitor of protein kinase C. In a small open study, tamoxifen appeared to have antimanic properties (Manji et al. 1999). If a mood-stabilizing action of tamoxifen were to be demonstrated in larger controlled trials, it could be a useful adjunct in the treatment of refractory bipolar disorder. However, adverse effects of this medication (for example, it precipitates menopause and increases the risk of uterine cancer) would make it appropriate only for life-threatening refractory illness. Mixed estrogen agonist/antagonist medications such as raloxifene have not been investigated as potential mood-stabilizing agents.

Mexiletine, an antiarrhythmic medication with anticonvulsant and analgesic properties, was studied in an open-label protocol involving patients with rapid-cycling bipolar disorder who could not tolerate lithium, valproate, or carbamazepine (Schaffer et al. 2000). A little less than half (46%) of the 20 patients who completed the study responded, and 15% had partial responses (defined as 25%–49% improvement on an overall rating of affective symptoms). No further information about applications of this medication in mood disorders is available.

In an open study involving 16 patients with bipolar depression and/or rapid cycling that was refractory to treatment with lithium, carbamazepine, divalproex, other anticonvulsants, and antidepressants, seven patients (44%) given the carbonic anhydrase inhibitor acetazolamide as an added agent had responses or remissions lasting as long as 2 years (Hayes 2001). No controlled studies of this medication have been performed.

A few case reports suggest that altering the timing of sleep and awakening may be a useful adjunct in the treatment of rapid cycling. One approach involves a "long night," in which the patient remains in bed in complete darkness for 10–14 hours. In addition to long nights for several weeks, the treatment entails 30 minutes of artificial bright light (10,000 lux) each morning, along with a walk outside for natural light therapy. Morning bright light has also been used without enforced sleep to stabilize the sleep–wake cycle and treat depression in patients with refractory rapid cycling. Because bright light is a potent zeitgeber, combining a sedating antipsychotic drug or a benzodiazepine at night with exposure to artificial bright light in the morning can help to reset the sleep–wake cycle and contribute to mood stabilization in patients with very unstable moods and erratic sleep. However, if the duration of bright light exposure is too long, hypomania and more mood cycling may result.

Stereotactic subcaudate tractotomy (SST), which involves precise localization of a lesion beneath the caudate nucleus, has been found in unstructured follow-up to benefit 50%–60% of the small number of patients with refractory bipolar disorder who have undergone this procedure (Bridges et al. 1994). The two study cohorts had 9 patients each, all of whom had continuous cycling refractory to all treatments. Patients were followed carefully for 2–13 years after undergoing SST. Three patients were essentially well and required no further treatment; 1 patient had mild residual symptoms; 11 patients continued to have affective episodes, but the episodes were less severe; 1 patient's condition was unchanged; and 2 patients had committed suicide. Like mood-stabilizing medications, SST was more effective for hypomania than depression. Complications of surgery included cognitive deficits in a few patients, schizophreniform symptoms in 1 patient, and partial relapse over time after initial improvement with surgery in several patients.

■ REFERENCES

Afflelou S, Auriacombe M, Cazenave M, et al: High dose levothyroxine for treatment of rapid cycling bipolar disorder: review of the literature and application to 6 subjects. Encephale 23:209–217, 1997

Altshuler LL, Keck PE Jr, McElroy SL, et al: Gabapentin in the acute treatment of refractory bipolar disorder. Bipolar Disord 1:61–65, 1999

American Psychiatric Association: Diagnostic and Statistical Manual of Mental Disorders, 4th Edition. Washington, DC, American Psychiatric Association, 1994

Anton RF, Burch EA: Response of psychotic depression subtypes to pharmacotherapy. J Affect Disord 28:125–131, 1993

Avissar S, Schreiber G: Interaction of antibipolar and antidepressant treatments with receptor-coupled G proteins. Pharmacopsychiatry 25 (1): 44–50, 1992

Baldessarini RJ, Tondo L, Floris G, et al: Effects of rapid cycling on response to lithium maintenance treatment in 360 bipolar I and II disorder patients. J Affect Disord 61:13–22, 2000

Barton BM, Gitlin MJ: Verapamil in treatment-resistant mania: an open trial. J Clin Psychopharmacol 7:101–103, 1987

Bauer MS, Whybrow PC: Rapid cycling bipolar affective disorder. Arch Gen Psychiatry 47:435–440, 1990

Bell KM, Potkin SG, Carreon D, et al: S-Adenosylmethionine blood levels in major depression: changes with drug treatment. Acta Neurol Scand Suppl 154:15–18, 1994

Ben-Shachar D, Gazawi H, Riboyad-Levin J, et al: Chronic repetitive transcranial magnetic stimulation alters beta-adrenergic and 5-HT$_2$ receptor characteristics in rat brain. Brain Res 816:78–83, 1999

Berghofer A, Muller-Oerlinghausen B: Is there a loss of efficacy of lithium in patients treated for over 20 years? Neuropsychobiology 42 (suppl 1):46–49, 2000

Berk M: Lamotrigine and the treatment of mania in bipolar disorder. Eur Neuropsychopharmacol 9:119–123, 1999

Berk M, Ichim L, Brook L: Olanzapine compared to lithium in mania: a double-blind randomized controlled trial. Int Clin Psychopharmacol 14:339–342, 1999

Bernstein L: Abrupt cessation of rapid-cycling bipolar disorder with the addition of low-dose L-tetraiodothyronine to lithium. J Clin Psychopharmacol 12:443–444, 1992

Black DW, Winokur G, Nasrallah A: Treatment of mania: a naturalistic study of electroconvulsive therapy versus lithium in 438 patients. J Clin Psychiatry 48:132–139, 1987

Bowden CL: Predictors of response to divalproex and lithium. J Clin Psychiatry 56 (suppl 3):25–30, 1995

Bowden CL, Brugger AM, Swann AC, et al: Efficacy of divalproex vs lithium and placebo in the treatment of mania. The Depakote Mania Study Group. JAMA 271:918–924, 1994

Bowden CL, Calabrese JR, McElroy SL, et al: The efficacy of lamotrigine in rapid cycling and non-rapid cycling patients with bipolar disorder. Biol Psychiatry 45:953–958, 1999

Bowden CL, Calabrese JR, Rapaport M, et al: Lamotrigine demonstrates long term mood stabilization in recently manic patients. Paper presented at the annual meeting of the NCDEU, May 2001

Bridges PK, Bartlett JR, Hale AS, et al: Psychosurgery: stereotactic subcaudate tractotomy. An indispensable treatment. Br J Psychiatry 165:599–611, 1994

Burke MJ, Preskhorn SH: Short-term treatment of mood disorders with standard antidepressants, in Psychopharmacology: The Fourth Generation of Progress. Edited by Bloom FE, Kupfer DJ. New York, Raven, 1995, pp 1053–1065

Burt T, Sachs GS, Demopulos C: Donepezil in treatment-resistant bipolar disorder. Biol Psychiatry 45 (8):959–964, 1999

Calabrese JR, Bowden CL, Sachs GS, et al: A double-blind placebo-controlled study of lamotrigine monotherapy in outpatients with bipolar I depression. Lamictal 602 Study Group. J Clin Psychiatry 60:79–88, 1999a

Calabrese JR, Bowden CL, McElroy SL, et al: Spectrum of activity of lamotrigine in treatment-refractory bipolar disorder. Am J Psychiatry 156:1019–1023, 1999b

Calabrese JR, Suppes T, Bowden CL, et al: A double-blind, placebo-controlled, prophylaxis study of lamotrigine in rapid-cycling bipolar disorder. Lamictal 614 Study Group. J Clin Psychiatry 61:841–850, 2000

Chengappa KN, Levine J, Gershon S, et al: Inositol as an add-on treatment for bipolar depression. Bipolar Disord 2:47–55, 2000

Coffey CE, Weiner RD, Djang WT, et al: Brain anatomic effects of electroconvulsive therapy: a prospective magnetic resonance imaging study. Arch Gen Psychiatry 48:1013–1017, 1991

Cozza KL, Armstrong SC: Concise Guide to the Cytochrome P450 System: Drug Interaction Principles for Medical Practice (Concise Guides). Washington, DC, American Psychiatric Publishing, 2001

Davanzo PA, Krah N, Kleiner J, et al: Nimodipine treatment of an adolescent with ultradian cycling bipolar affective illness. J Child Adolesc Psychopharmacol 9:51–61, 1999

Devanand DP, Sackeim HA, Prudic J: Electroconvulsive therapy in the treatment-resistant patient. Psychiatr Clin North Am 14:905–923, 1991

Dietrich DE, Kropp S, Emrich HM: Oxcarbazepine in affective and schizoaffective disorders. Pharmacopsychiatry 34 (6):242–250, 2001

Doris A, Ebmeier KP, Shajahan P: Depressive illness. Lancet 354:1369–1375, 1999

Dubovsky SL: Electroconvulsive therapy, in Comprehensive Textbook of Psychiatry/VI, 6th Edition, Vol 2. Edited by Kaplan HI, Sadock BJ. Baltimore, MD, Williams & Wilkins, 1995, pp 2129–2140

Dubovsky SL, Thomas M: Tardive dyskinesia associated with fluoxetine. Psychiatr Serv 47:991–993, 1996

Dubovsky SL, Franks RD, Allen S, et al: Calcium antagonists in mania: a double-blind study of verapamil. Psychiatry Res 18:309–320, 1986

Dwight MM, Keck PE, Jr, Stanton SP, et al: Antidepressant activity and mania associated with risperidone treatment of schizoaffective disorder. Lancet 344:554–555, 1994

Elkin I, Shea MT, Watkins JT, et al: National Institute of Mental Health Treatment of Depression Collaborative Research Program: general effectiveness of treatments. Arch Gen Psychiatry 46 (11):971–982, 1989

Expert Consensus Panel for Bipolar Disorder: Treatment of bipolar disorder. J Clin Psychiatry 57 (suppl 12A):3–88, 1996

Frye MA, Ketter TA, Kimbrell TA, et al: A placebo-controlled study of lamotrigine and gabapentin monotherapy in refractory mood disorders. J Clin Psychopharmacol 20:607–614, 2000

Gaster B, Holroyd J: St John's wort for depression: a systematic review. Arch Intern Med 160 (2):152–156, 2001

Gelenberg AJ, Kane JM, Keller MB, et al: Comparison of standard and low serum levels of lithium for maintenance treatment of bipolar disorder. N Engl J Med 321:1489–1493, 1989

George MS, Wassermann EM, Kimbrell TA, et al: Mood improvement following daily left prefrontal repetitive transcranial magnetic stimulation in patients with depression: a placebo-controlled crossover trial. Am J Psychiatry 154:1752–1756, 1997

Gershon S, Soares JC: Current therapeutic profile of lithium. Arch Gen Psychiatry 54:16–18, 1997

Ghaemi SN, Goodwin FK: Use of atypical antipsychotic agents in bipolar and schizoaffective disorders: review of the empirical literature. J Clin Psychopharmacol 19:354–361, 1999

Gjessing LR: Disturbances of somatic function in catatonia with a periodic course and their compensation. J Ment Sci 84:608–621, 1938

Glassman A, Preud'homme XA: Review of the cardiovascular effects of heterocyclic antidepressants. J Clin Psychiatry 54 (suppl):16–22, 1993

Goldberg JF, Harrow M, Leon AC: Lithium treatment of bipolar affective disorders under naturalistic followup conditions. Psychopharmacol Bull 32:47–54, 1996

Goodnick PJ: Verapamil prophylaxis in pregnant women with bipolar disorder (letter). Am J Psychiatry 150:1560, 1993

Green AI, Tohen M, Patel JK, et al: Clozapine in the treatment of refractory psychotic mania. Am J Psychiatry 157:982–986, 2000

Grisaru N, Chudakov B, Yaroslavsky Y, et al: Transcranial magnetic stimulation in mania: a controlled study. Am J Psychiatry 155:1608–1610, 1998

Haddjeri N, Blier P: Sustained blockade of neurokinin-1 receptors enhances serotonin neurotransmission. Biol Psychiatry 50 (3):191–199, 2001

Hayes SG: Acetazolamide in bipolar affective disorders. Ann Clin Psychiatry 6:91–98, 2001

Hopkins HS, Gelenberg AJ: Treatment of bipolar disorder: how far have we come? Psychopharmacol Bull 30:27–38, 1994

Hoshino M, Heise CO, Puglia P, et al: Hepatic enzymes' level during chronic use of anticonvulsant drugs. Arq Neuropsiquiatr 53:719–723, 1995

Isojarvi JI, Laatikainen TJ, Pakarinen AJ, et al: Polycystic ovaries and hyperandrogenism in women taking valproate for epilepsy. N Engl J Med 329:1383–1388, 1993

Janicak PG, Sharma RP, Pandey G, et al: Verapamil for the treatment of acute mania: a double-blind, placebo-controlled trial. Am J Psychiatry 155 (7): 972–973, 1998

Kato M, Katayama T, Iwata H, et al: In vivo characterization of T-794, a novel reversible inhibitor of monoamine oxidase-A, as an antidepressant with a wide safety margin. J Pharmacol Exp Ther 284:983–990, 1998

Keck PE Jr, McElroy SL, Tugrul KC, et al: Valproate oral loading in the treatment of acute mania. J Clin Psychiatry 54:305–308, 1993

Keck PE Jr, McElroy SL, Strakowski SM, et al: Factors associated with pharmacologic noncompliance in patients with mania. J Clin Psychiatry 57 (7):292–297, 1996

Kleindienst N, Greil W: Differential efficacy of lithium and carbamazepine in the prophylaxis of bipolar disorder: results of the MAP study. Neuropsychobiology 42 (suppl 1):2–10, 2000

Kocsis JH, Frances AJ, Voss C, et al: Imipramine treatment for chronic depression. Arch Gen Psychiatry 45:253–257, 1988

Labbate LA, Lafer B, Thibault A, et al: Influence of phototherapy treatment duration for seasonal affective disorder: outcome at one vs. two weeks. Biol Psychiatry 38:747–750, 1995

Lee DO, Steingard RJ, Cesena M, et al: Behavioral side effects of gabapentin in children. Epilepsia 37:87–90, 1996

Levine J, Barak Y, Gonzalves M, et al: Double-blind, controlled trial of inositol treatment of depression. Am J Psychiatry 152:792–794, 1995

Leweke FM, Bauer J, Elger CE: Manic episode due to gabapentin treatment (letter). Br J Psychiatry 175:291, 1999

Licht RW: Drug treatment of mania: a critical review. Acta Psychiatr Scand 97:387–397, 1998

Lieb K, Fiebich BL, Berger M: [Substance P receptor antagonists: a new antidepressive and anxiolytic mechanism?] Nervenarzt 71 (9):758–761, 2000

Lindhout D, Omtzigt JG: Pregnancy and the risk of teratogenicity. Epilepsia 33 (suppl 4):S41–S48, 1992

Loo C, Mitchell P, Sachdev P, et al: Double-blind controlled investigation of transcranial magnetic stimulation for the treatment of resistant major depression. Am J Psychiatry 156:946–948, 1999

Manji HK, Bebchuk JM, Moore GJ, et al: Modulation of CNS signal transduction pathways and gene expression by mood-stabilizing agents: therapeutic implications. J Clin Psychiatry 60 (suppl 2):27–39, 1999

Manna V: Disturbi affettivi bipolari e ruolo del calcio intraneuronale: effetti terapeutici del trattamento con cali di litio e/o calcio antagonista in pazienti con rapida inversione di polarita. Minerva Med 82:757–763, 1991

Marder SR: Atypical antipsychotic agents in the treatment of schizophrenia and other psychiatric disorders, part I: unique patient populations. J Clin Psychiatry 59:259–265, 1998

McElroy SL, Keck PE Jr, Strakowski SM: Mania, psychosis, and antipsychotics. J Clin Psychiatry 57 (suppl 3):14–26, 1996

McElroy SL, Suppes T, Keck PE, et al: Open-label adjunctive topiramate in the treatment of bipolar disorders. Biol Psychiatry 47:1025–1033, 2000

Miller RJ, Chouinard G: Loss of striatal cholinergic neurons as a basis for tardive and L-dopa-induced dyskinesias, neuroleptic-induced supersensitivity psychosis and refractory schizophrenia. Biol Psychiatry 34:713–738, 1993

Mosimann UP, Rihs TA, Engeler J, et al: Mood effects of repetitive transcranial magnetic stimulation of left prefrontal cortex in healthy volunteers. Psychiatry Res 94:252–256, 2000

Mosolov SN, Moshchevitin SL: Use of electroconvulsive therapy for breaking the continuous course of drug-resistant affective and schizoaffective psychoses. Zhurnal Nevropatologii i Psikhiatrii Imeni S.S. Korsakova 90:121–125, 1990

Murphy BE: Antiglucocorticoid therapies in major depression: a review. Psychoneuroendocrinology 22 (suppl 1):S125–S132, 1997

Murphy BE, Filipini D, Ghadirian AM: Possible use of glucocorticoid receptor antagonists in the treatment of major depression: preliminary results using RU-486. J Psychiatry Neurosci 18:209–213, 1995

Mukherjee S, Sackeim HA, Schnur DB: Electroconvulsive therapy of acute manic episodes: a review of 50 years' experience. Am J Psychiatry 151:169–176, 1994

Nemets B, Mishory A, Levine J, et al: Inositol addition does not improve depression in SSRI treatment failures. J Neural Transm 106:795–798, 1999

Okuma T: Effects of carbamazepine and lithium on affective disorders. Neuropsychobiology 27:138–145, 1993

Okuma T, Yamashita I, Takahashi R, et al: Comparison of the antimanic efficacy of carbamazepine and lithium carbonate by double-blind controlled study. Pharmacopsychiatry 23:143–150, 1990

Pande AC, Crockatt JG, Janney CA, et al: Gabapentin in bipolar disorder: a placebo-controlled trial of adjunctive therapy. Gabapentin Bipolar Disorder Study Group. Bipolar Disord 2:249–255, 2000

Partonen T, Sihvo S, Lonnqvist JK: Patients excluded from an antidepressant efficacy trial. J Clin Psychiatry 57:572–575, 1996

Pazzaglia PJ, Post RM, Ketter TA, et al: Preliminary controlled trial of nimodipine in ultra-rapid cycling affective dysregulation. Psychiatry Res 49:257–272, 1993

Peet M, Murphy B, Shay J, et al: Depletion of omega-3 fatty acid levels in red blood cell membranes of depressive patients. Biol Psychiatry 43:315–319, 1998

Perry PJ, Zeilmann C, Arndt S: Tricyclic antidepressant concentrations in plasma: an estimate of their sensitivity and specificity as a predictor of response. J Clin Psychopharmacol 14:230–235, 1994

Post RM: Prophylaxis of bipolar affective disorders. International Review of Psychiatry 2:277–320, 1990

Prange AJJ: Novel uses of thyroid hormones in patients with affective disorders. Thyroid 6:537–543, 1996

Reeves RR: Does EEG predict response to valproate versus lithium in patients with mania? Ann Clin Psychiatry 13:69–73, 2001

Rosenthal NE, Oren DA: Light therapy, in Treatments of Psychiatric Disorders, 2nd Edition. Edited by Gabbard GO. Washington, DC, American Psychiatric Press, 1995, pp 1263–1273

Rupniak NM: Elucidating the antidepressant actions of substance P (NK1 receptor) antagonists. Curr Opin Investig Drugs 3 (2):257–261, 2002

Sachs GS, Printz DJ, Kahn DA, et al: The Expert Consensus Guideline Series: medication treatment of bipolar disorder 2000. Postgrad Med (Spec No):1–104, 2000

Saxena S, Mallikarjuna P: Severe memory impairment with acute overdose lithium toxicity: a case report. Br J Psychiatry 152:853–854, 1988

Schaffer A, Levitt AJ, Joffe RT: Mexiletine in treatment-resistant bipolar disorder. J Affect Disord 57:249–253, 2000

Schatzberg AF, Nemeroff CB (eds): American Psychiatric Press Textbook of Psychopharmacology, 2nd Edition. Washington, DC, American Psychiatric Press, 1998

Schnur DB, Mukherjee S, Sackeim HA, et al: Symptomatic predictors of ECT response in medication-nonresponsive manic patients. J Clin Psychiatry 53:63–66, 1992

Sernyak MJ, Woods SW: Chronic neuroleptic use in manic-depressive illness. Psychopharmacol Bull 29:375–381, 1993

Shelton RC, Keller MB, Gelenberg AJ, et al: Effectiveness of St. John's wort in major depression: a randomized controlled trial. JAMA 285:1978–1986, 2001a

Shelton RC, Tollefson GD, Tohen M, et al: A novel augmentation strategy for treating resistant major depression. Am J Psychiatry 158:131–134, 2001b

Simon AE, Aubry JM, Malky L, et al: Hypomania-like syndrome induced by olanzapine. Int Clin Psychopharmacol 14:377–378, 1999

Small JG, Klapper MH, Milstein V, et al: Comparison of therapeutic modalities for mania. Psychopharmacol Bull 32:623–627, 1996

Sporn J, Ghaemi SN, Rankin MA, et al: Pramipexole augmentation in the treatment of unipolar and bipolar depression: a retrospective chart review. Ann Clin Psychiatry 12:137–140, 2000

Stancer HC, Persad E: Treatment of intractable rapid-cycling manic-depressive disorder with levothyroxine: clinical observations. Arch Gen Psychiatry 39:311–312, 1982

Stoll AL, Severus WE, Freeman MP, et al: Omega 3 fatty acids in bipolar disorder: a preliminary double-blind, placebo-controlled trial. Arch Gen Psychiatry 56:407–412, 1999

Suppes T, Webb A, Paul B, et al: Clinical outcome in a randomized 1-year trial of clozapine versus treatment as usual for patients with treatment-resistant illness and a history of mania. Am J Psychiatry 156:1164–1169, 1999

Swoboda E, Conca A, Konig P, et al: Maintenance electroconvulsive therapy in affective and schizoaffective disorder. Neuropsychobiology 43:23–28, 2001

Tam EM, Lam RWA, Levitt AJ: Treatment of seasonal affective disorder: a review. Can J Psychiatry 40:457–466, 1995

Tohen M, Sanger TM, McElroy SL, et al: Olanzapine versus placebo in the treatment of acute mania. Am J Psychiatry 156:702–709, 1999

Tohen M, Jacobs TG, Grundy SL, et al: Efficacy of olanzapine in acute bipolar mania: a double-blind, placebo-controlled study. The Olanzapine HGGW Study Group. Arch Gen Psychiatry 57:841–849, 2000

Tohen M, Baker RW, Altschuler LL, et al: Olanzapine versus divalproex in the treatment of acute mania. Am J Psychiatry 159 (6):1011–1017, 2002

Vestergaard P, Licht RW, Brodersen A, et al: Outcome of lithium prophylaxis: a prospective follow-up of affective disorder patients assigned to high and low serum lithium levels. Acta Psychiatr Scand 98:310–315, 1998

Vieta E, Reinares M, Corbella B, et al: Olanzapine as long-term adjunctive therapy in treatment-resistant bipolar disorder. J Clin Psychopharmacol 21 (5):469–473, 2001

Walden J, Schaerer L, Schloesser S, et al: An open longitudinal study of patients with bipolar rapid cycling treated with lithium or lamotrigine for mood stabilization. Bipolar Disord 2:336–339, 2000

Willoughby CL, Hradek EA, Richards NR: Use of electroconvulsive therapy with children: an overview and case report. J Child Adolesc Psychiatr Nurs 10:11–17, 1997

Wisner KL, Peindl KS, Perel JM, et al: Verapamil treatment for women with bipolar disorder. Biol Psychiatry 51 (9):745–752, 2002

Woelk H: Comparison of St John's wort and imipramine for treating depression: randomised controlled trial. BMJ 321:536–539, 2000

Wolkowitz OD, Reus VI: Treatment of depression with antiglucocorticoid drugs. Psychosom Med 61:698–711, 1999

Wolpert EA, Berman E, Bernstein M: Efficacy of electroconvulsive therapy in continuous rapid cycling bipolar disorder. Psychiatric Annals 29: 679–683, 1999

5

PSYCHOTHERAPIES FOR MOOD DISORDERS

Administration of antidepressant medications has become an important treatment for unipolar depression. In one report, Roose and Stern (1995) noted that 29% of 56 patients in psychoanalysis with analytic candidates were taking these medications. However, a number of psychotherapies have been found to be as effective as antidepressants, especially in less severe cases of unipolar depression. Two psychotherapies designed specifically for major depression— cognitive therapy (CT) (and a variant, cognitive-behavioral therapy [CBT]) and interpersonal psychotherapy (IPT)—have been subjected to controlled research and have been compared with treatment with reference antidepressants. However, these studies have several features that complicate interpretation of the results. For example, most psychotherapy studies have involved patients with mild to moderate nonpsychotic unipolar depression. In addition, many comparisons of psychotherapy and pharmacotherapy used imipramine, the standard reference antidepressant, in a fixed-dose protocol. The dropout rate among imipramine-treated patients in such protocols is greater than among patients taking antidepressants in clinical practice, where better-tolerated antidepressants are used and components of pharmacotherapy include encouraging compliance and adjusting the dose as necessary. In addition, antidepressants and psychotherapies may not be directly comparable because they act on different symptoms: psychotherapy works faster to improve social function and suicidal thinking, whereas medications bring about earlier improvement of mood, sleep, and appetite.

In the National Institute of Mental Health multicenter collaborative study of treatments for depression, patients with nonpsychotic unipolar depression underwent a 16-week course of IPT, CBT, placebo plus "clinical management" (nonspecific supportive psychotherapy), or imipramine therapy plus clinical management (Elkin et al. 1989). For mildly depressed patients, no active treatment was any more effective than placebo plus clinical management, probably reflecting a high rate of spontaneous improvement or at least fluctuation of symptoms in this population. As depression became more severe, imipramine plus clinical management was found to be consistently superior on the broadest range of outcome measures. IPT was better than placebo but not as effective as imipramine. CBT was only slightly less effective than IPT, but it was not significantly better than placebo. The results suggested that support and no medication might be effective for mild acute depression, whereas more severely depressed patients appear to require antidepressants.

This conclusion is not as straightforward as it might seem. The method of analysis involving the last observation carried forward may have underestimated the efficacy of both psychotherapies, and other research suggests that cognitive-behavioral psychotherapy and IPT are effective for severe depression (Jarrett 1997). However, IPT and behavior therapy may be less effective in melancholic than in nonmelancholic depression. Relapse of depression does not occur as rapidly after discontinuation of psychotherapy as it does after withdrawal of antidepressants, and continuation of psychotherapy after recovery reduces the relapse rate (Thase and Kupfer 1996), as does continuation of antidepressant therapy after recovery. In clinical practice, most patients benefit from combinations of medications and psychotherapy (discussed in "Combined Treatment: Pharmacotherapy and Psychotherapy").

■ COGNITIVE THERAPY

CT is based on the premise that the negative emotions of depression are reactions to negative thinking derived from dysfunctional global negative attitudes. Patient and therapist work together to identify automatic negative thoughts, correct the pervasive beliefs that generate these thoughts, and develop more realistic basic assumptions. Treatment involves systematically monitoring negative cognitions whenever the patient feels depressed; recognizing the association between cognition, affect, and behavior; generating data that support or refute the negative cognition; generating alternative hypotheses to explain the event that precipitated the negative cognition; and identifying the negative schemata predisposing to the emergence of global negative thinking when one side of an all-or-nothing assumption is disappointed. In the course of examining dysfunctional attitudes, the patient learns to label and counteract information-processing errors such as overgeneralization, excessive personalization, all-or-nothing thinking, and generalization from single negative events.

For example, after keeping track of what he was thinking at the moment he began to feel depressed, a man might realize that the feeling started after he began thinking "nobody loves me" when his wife did not greet him enthusiastically after work. This thought might be seen to follow logically from the assumption "If she isn't always happy to see me, she doesn't love me." Two kinds of alternative hypotheses could be generated in considering this cognition. First, the patient's wife may have been preoccupied, or it may be that she was happy to see him but did not demonstrate it in exactly the way he expected. Second, lack of enthusiasm at one particular moment is not necessarily a sign of generalized disinterest. Eventually, the patient learns to correct the underlying all-or-nothing belief that "people either are completely devoted to me or they don't care at all."

The best studied of the psychotherapies for major depression, CT has been compared with nonpharmacological control conditions as acute treatment for depression in at least 21 randomized controlled clinical trials. In a meta-analysis of 12 suitable studies, CT had an overall efficacy rate of 46.6% and was 30.1% more effective than no therapy when the control was a waiting list (two studies), but CT was only 9.4% more effective than placebo plus clinical management in the collaborative study mentioned early in the chapter (Elkin et al. 1989). Although CT was demonstrated in early studies to be superior to pharmacotherapy provided by a primary care physician, comparisons with more rigorous pharmacological treatment provided by psychiatrists suggest that the two treatments are equally effective for depression of moderate severity (Hollon et al. 1992). Modified CT was shown to be effective for hospitalized depressed patients (Stuart and Thase 1994). Pharmacotherapy was more effective than CT in more severely depressed patients in the National Institute of Mental Health collaborative study (Elkin et al. 1989). The onset of action of antidepressants has been found to be faster than the onset of action of CT.

Some studies suggest that starting treatment with an antidepressant and then adding CT (sequential combined therapy) may be more effective than adding antidepressants to CT (Hollon et al. 1992), presumably because residual symptoms after a response to an antidepressant are more responsive to CT than residual symptoms after a partial response to CT and to antidepressants. However, in clinical practice, patients with poor responses to CT (or any psychotherapy) alone often respond to the addition of antidepressants. Rates of response to individual CT exceed rates of response to group CT (50.1% vs. 39.2%) (Thase and Kupfer 1996). Depressed patients with personality disorders may be more likely to drop out of CT, but those who remain in treatment can improve as much as patients without Axis II disorders.

Monthly CT achieved the same level of prophylaxis as continuation pharmacotherapy in one study (Blackburn et al. 1986). In a naturalistic follow-up study involving patients who responded to CT, patients who responded to antidepressants and were then withdrawn from medication, and patients who responded to antidepressants and received continuation pharmacotherapy, CT-treated patients relapsed significantly less often than patients who were no longer receiving antidepressant monotherapy (21% vs. 50% at 2 years); the relapse rate for maintenance CT was comparable to that for maintenance antidepressant therapy (15%) (Evans et al. 1992).

Following successful treatment with antidepressant medication, CBT was shown to reduce the risk of relapse of unipolar depression, at least in the relatively near term, after withdrawal of the antidepressant (Thase 1992). After recovering from at least a third episode of major depression, for which tricyclics or selective serotonin reuptake inhibitors were administered according to a standardized protocol similar to that used in a study by Frank et al. (1990), 40 patients continued taking full doses of antidepressants for 3–5 months. At the end of this period, patients were randomly assigned to pharmacotherapy plus CBT or pharmacotherapy plus clinical management. Antidepressants were then withdrawn at a rate of 25 mg of amitriptyline equivalent every other week. All patients were medication free during the last 2 CBT sessions. CBT included treatment of residual negative cognitions, exposure to reduce anxiety, lifestyle modification, and well-being therapy (a 2- to 3-session approach to changing attitudes that interfere with positive self-regard, relationships with others, environmental mastery, and personal growth). Patients were followed for 2 years after CBT was completed.

In this study, CBT but not clinical management resulted in significant improvement of residual symptoms and one-third the risk of relapse over the 2 years of treatment-free follow-up. After another 4 years (i.e., 6 years after completion of CBT), patients who had been treated with CBT had fewer relapses, although they were as likely to have at least one relapse as those who had had clinical management. Of course, the question of whether simply continuing antidepressant therapy would have had a similar prophylactic effect was not addressed. The authors speculated that the short course of CBT (10 vs. the usual 16–20 sessions) was effective because CBT was added after medications had established a remission, at which point CBT was needed only for residual symptoms that might predispose to relapse.

■ INTERPERSONAL PSYCHOTHERAPY

IPT is designed to improve depression by enhancing the quality of the patient's interpersonal world. The treatment begins with an explanation of the diagnosis and treatment options; this first step serves to legitimate depression as a medical illness. The acute course of treatment is conducted according to a manual-based protocol over 12–16 weeks. A protocol for maintenance IPT has also been developed. Through structured assignments, IPT helps the patient to work toward explicit goals related to whichever of the four basic interpersonal problems (unresolved grief, role disputes, transitions to new roles, and social skills deficits) is believed to be important. Role-playing is used to help the patient acquire new interpersonal skills, and structured conjoint meetings are used to help partners clarify their expectations of each other.

Some clinicians believe that IPT is no more than a specialized form of expressive (psychodynamic) psychotherapy, but there are important differences between the two treatments. Unlike expressive psychotherapy, IPT follows a structured approach outlined in a manual and involves explicit homework assignments. Its focus is exclusively on the present; there is no systematic attempt to explore conflicts related to early experience, to address transference, or to change underlying character structure. IPT may be a more acceptable pharmacotherapy or cognitive or behavioral therapy, at least to younger patients.

In initial randomized clinical trials involving outpatients with nonpsychotic major depression, IPT was superior to amitriptyline in producing improvement in mood, suicidal ideation, and interest, whereas the antidepressant was more effective for appetite and sleep disturbances (Thase 1995). In a comparison with nortriptyline in older patients, IPT was found to be as effective in reducing depressive symptoms, and more IPT-treated patients than nortriptyline-treated patients remained in the study. In the collaborative study (described early in the chapter) comparing IPT, CT, imipramine therapy plus clinical management, and placebo plus clinical management, IPT was found to be equivalent to imipramine therapy and CT by the end of 16 weeks, but imipramine was more rapidly effective (Elkin et al. 1989).

IPT has been shown to be effective as maintenance treatment as well as acute therapy. In a prospective study involving 128 patients, each of whom had had at least two previous episodes of recurrent unipolar depression, patients were randomized to one of five treatment conditions after achieving remission through acute treatment with imipramine: monthly IPT plus imipramine, monthly IPT plus placebo, monthly IPT alone, imipramine plus supportive management, or placebo plus supportive management (Frank et al. 1990). The active-medication conditions were associated with relapse-free rates of roughly 80% at 3-year follow-up. In addition, at 3 years, IPT with or without placebo had more than doubled relapse-free survival rates compared with placebo and supportive care (30%–40% vs. 10%). Blind independent ratings of the quality of IPT demonstrated that patients treated with higher-quality IPT had relapse-free survival rates comparable to rates among patients treated with imipramine. Patients receiving IPT of below-average quality had survival rates that were no better than rates among patients receiving placebo (Frank et al. 1991).

In a subsequent study, 20 patients who had been treated with imipramine and had remained in remission for the first 3 years of the first study (Frank et al. 1990) were randomized to 2 years of continued treatment with the antidepressant or 2 years of placebo (Kupfer et al. 1992). Eighty-two percent of those treated with medication survived the next 2 years without a depressive recurrence, compared with 33% of those randomized to placebo. Only 11% of those receiving placebo alone survived, whereas 78% of patients in the first study who continued with monthly IPT and placebo remained relapse-free. Not investigated was the possibility that a maintenance IPT "dose" greater than the monthly sessions used in these studies might have produced even better results.

IPT was an effective adjunct to maintenance antidepressant therapy in elderly patients in one study (Reynolds et al. 1995). Another study involved 180 geriatric patients with recurrent nonpsychotic unipolar depression who were experiencing at least a second lifetime episode of unipolar depression after having been well for 3 years or less (Flint and Rifat 1996). Patients were treated openly with weekly IPT and nortriptyline (serum level, 0–120 ng/mL), with or without lithium or perphenazine augmentation, until depression remitted (Hamilton Rating Scale for Depression score of 10 or less). Patients were then treated for 16 weeks to ensure stability of remission, after which the 107 patients whose remissions remained stable were randomly assigned to medication clinic plus nortriptyline; medication clinic plus placebo; monthly IPT plus nortriptyline; or monthly IPT plus placebo. Patients continued maintenance treatment for 3 years or until recurrence of major depression. All active treatments were significantly better than placebo in preventing recurrence. Combined IPT and nortriptyline therapy was superior to IPT plus placebo (recurrence rate over 3 years, 20% vs. 64%). The combination of IPT and the antidepressant was most effective in preventing recurrences during the first year of maintenance, because this was when most recurrences took place, especially in patients older than 70 years.

A form of IPT called *interpersonal and social rhythm therapy* (IPSRT) is under study as an adjunct to thymoleptic medication therapy in the maintenance treatment of bipolar mood disorders. In addition to interpersonal techniques such as resolving interpersonal conflicts and encouraging the expression of grief for the loss of the person the patient was before the illness began, IPSRT includes a structured approach to normalizing circadian rhythms. The patient first keeps a log of the timing of 17 zeitgebers (e.g., getting out of bed, meals, first interaction with another person, exercising, going to bed). Average times are computed for each of these cues to circadian rhythms, and the patient is helped to keep a regular schedule for each of them.

After 1 year of prospective comparison of IPSRT and supportive psychotherapy (an education and medication-compliance module was used; each psychotherapy was added to standard pharmacotherapy protocols) in patients who had achieved remission of mania or bipolar depression for at least 4 months, Frank et al. (1997) noted that patients treated with IPSRT were significantly more likely to have normalized their schedules of the 17 circadian cues (i.e., their schedules were identical to those of control populations studied with the same instrument). There were no significant clinical differences between the IPSRT and supportive psychotherapy groups after half of this planned 2-year study in a relatively small population had been completed. However, determining the benefit of IPSRT as an adjunctive maintenance treatment probably will require studying large samples over longer periods, to control for variance in illness and treatment.

■ FAMILY THERAPY

Involvement of the family is a defining characteristic of IPT. Family-focused treatment is a manual-based psychoeducational treatment for bipolar disorder. The goals of this approach are to alter family interactions that interfere with medication adherence and to promote affective recurrences. Patients and their relatives are exposed to a series of modules that focus on educating patients and families about bipolar illness in general and patients' own symptoms in particular, developing a relapse prevention plan, enhancing communication between patients and their relatives, and solving family problems. A recent study demonstrated that family-focused treatment added to open treatment with mood-stabilizing medications was associated with fewer relapses and longer delays before relapses (Miklowitz et al. 2000). In everyday practice, family involvement is important for most patients with mood disorders, whether or not specific family therapies are employed.

■ BEHAVIOR THERAPY

Therapies for depression derived from principles of classic and operant conditioning, social learning theory, and learned helplessness include social learning approaches, self-control therapy, social skills training, and structured problem-solving therapy. Behavior therapies use education, guided practice, homework assignments, and social reinforcement of successive approximations of nondepressed behavior in a time-limited format, typically over 8–16 weeks. Depressive behaviors such as self-blame, passivity, and negativism are ignored, whereas behaviors that are inconsistent with depression, such as activity, experiencing pleasure, and solving problems, are rewarded. Rewards can be anything that the patient seems to seek out—from attention, to praise, to being permitted to withdraw or complain, to money. Giving the patient small, discrete tasks that very gradually become more demanding reverses learned helplessness. For example, the person who feels hopeless about finding a job is first given the task of getting a newspaper. The next task is merely to look at the want ads, and only later is a list of possible jobs drawn up and one letter of application written. Each positive experience reinforces a feeling of accomplishment that makes the next task easier. Social skills training teaches self-reinforcement, assertive behavior, and the use of social reinforcers such as eye contact and compliments.

In a meta-analysis of 10 suitable studies by the Agency for Health Care Policy and Research (1993), behavior therapy had an overall intention-to-treat efficacy rate of 55.3% and appeared to have a small advantage over comparison psychotherapies in six studies and pharmacotherapy in two studies. However, the adequacy of the treatments to which behavior therapy was compared has been questioned (Crits-Christoph 1992; Meterissian and Bradwejn 1989). Behavior therapy has appeared to be as effective in depression (Brown and Lewinsohn 1984) as in other psychiatric disorders (Budman et al. 1988). Group and individual behavior therapies seem to have similar efficacy rates.

Fewer studies have demonstrated that maintenance behavior therapy is effective in preventing depressive recurrence than have shown that behavior therapy is effective as an acute treatment (Thase 1995). However, some studies comparing behavior therapy with no psychotherapy suggest that the benefits of behavior therapy persist after treatment is discontinued (McLean and Hakstian 1990); other studies do not support this hypothesis (Gallagher-Thompson et al. 1990). Adding antidepressants to behavior therapy did not enhance outcome in three older randomized outpatient trials of the combination, but improvement was more rapid in two of these trials (Herson et al. 1984; Roth et al. 1982; Wilson 1982).

Antidepressants may also have helped a greater number of more severely depressed patients to remain in trials of behavior therapy.

■ PSYCHODYNAMIC PSYCHOTHERAPY

At one time, extended and often unstructured psychodynamic psychotherapy was the standard psychotherapy for depression, and some case reports seemed to indicate that it was effective for depression. With more experience, the utility of nondirective psychodynamic approaches as a treatment for depression (as opposed to character pathology) was increasingly questioned (Thase 1995). The question remains open because no controlled studies of prolonged psychodynamic psychotherapy or psychoanalysis in mood disorders have been conducted. However, it seems unlikely that a treatment that can take years could be shown to be better than other treatments for acute depression, which often remits without treatment in a shorter period. Studies of the effectiveness of prolonged expressive psychotherapy in resolving conflicts and attitudes that predispose to recurrence would have a better chance of success, but funding for such expensive studies is unlikely to be available.

Brief dynamic psychotherapies have been applied to depressive disorders, but they have not been studied as rigorously as have CT and IPT. Methodological deficiencies limit the ability to draw conclusions from eight randomized controlled trials of brief dynamic therapy in depression (Gabbard 1995). For example, low rates of response (approximately 35%) to both psychotherapy and treatment with antidepressants raise questions about the adequacy of either treatment and the nature of the samples. In addition, five of the eight studies examined dynamic psychotherapy in a group format, even though individual therapy is more widely practiced, and the therapy sessions were usually conducted by nonprofessional therapists who were not formally trained in brief dynamic therapy (Gabbard 1995). These scientific issues notwithstanding, gifted clinicians may find that dynamic psychotherapy is highly effective for depression, especially if the illness is chronic or complicated by character pathology.

■ MOTIVATIONAL ENHANCEMENT AND RELAPSE PREVENTION

Motivational enhancement, a manual-based therapy developed for the treatment of substance dependence, has been modified to serve as an adjunctive approach designed to enhance compliance with antidepressant therapy. Compliance is a particularly important problem in primary care practice, where few depressed patients continue taking antidepressants for the minimum recommended 6–9 months after remission of a single episode of major depression, and where even fewer receive longer-term maintenance treatment despite the high rate of relapse and recurrence. A relapse prevention program developed for primary care practices uses a version of motivational enhancement that includes development of an individualized treatment plan and a review of potential advantages and disadvantages of continuing antidepressant therapy; regular support; and outreach to patients with evidence of symptom return and to patients' primary physicians. This approach was tested in an efficacy study, which demonstrated that primary care patients randomly assigned to the relapse prevention program had greater medication adherence and fewer depressive symptoms but did not have a reduction in rates of relapse or recurrence over 1 year of follow-up (Katon et al. 2001).

■ CHARACTERISTICS OF EFFECTIVE PSYCHOTHERAPY FOR DEPRESSION

Even though data from controlled studies of psychotherapy of depression are limited, characteristics listed in Table 5–1 have repeatedly emerged as distinguishing effective treatments, regardless of the technical details of the therapy. Extended, unstructured psychotherapies may be useful for treating associated problems such as personality disorders and family dysfunction, but given the lack of data supporting the use of these therapies as primary treatments for depression, more focused, time-limited therapies seem appropriate

TABLE 5–1.	Characteristics of effective psychotherapy for depression

Time-limited treatment
Explicit rationale for treatment, shared by patient and therapist
Active and directive therapist
Focus on current problems
Emphasis on changing current behavior
Self-monitoring of progress
Involvement of significant others
Expression of cautious optimism
Problems divided into manageable units with short-term goals
Homework assignments

for primary depression, at least as initial approaches. When issues such as the effect of early trauma or abuse appear to be indications for longer-term psychotherapy, it may be more expedient to treat depression first and address other issues once depression has remitted. Emotionally charged material may be intensified by depression, making it more difficult to resolve. When the material proves overwhelming, the patient feels even more helpless and unsuccessful, and depression worsens.

■ COMBINED TREATMENT: PHARMACOTHERAPY AND PSYCHOTHERAPY

Hollon and Fawcett (1995) reviewed two studies of dynamic psychodynamic therapy, three trials of behavior therapy, and nine studies of CT. In all studies, antidepressants were added during the acute phase of treatment. The investigators found only a statistically insignificant trend toward superiority of combined treatment over each treatment by itself, mainly because the studies had insufficient statistical power. Until more informative data become available about mild to moderate nonpsychotic unipolar depression, it seems most reasonable to treat such episodes either with antidepressants or with one of the structured psychotherapies for depression.

Although psychotherapy and antidepressants are equally effective for mild depression, controlled, outpatient studies of nonbipolar depression show that combined pharmacotherapy and psychotherapy is significantly more effective than psychotherapy alone for severe depression. Thase et al. (1997) conducted a meta-analysis of original data from 595 patients with nonbipolar, nonpsychotic major depressive disorder who were treated for 16 weeks with either CBT or IPT alone ($n=243$) or IPT plus an antidepressant ($n=352$) (a total of six standardized treatment protocols were used). In mild depression, combined therapy was not significantly more effective than psychotherapy alone. However, in more severe recurrent major depression, combined treatment was significantly more effective. The combination of a form of cognitive behavior therapy and treatment with nefazodone was statistically and clinically significantly superior to either treatment alone in producing initial improvement and preventing relapse in patients with chronic depression (Keller et al. 2000).

Some experts suggest that more severe major depressive episodes be treated first with antidepressants alone, so that patients who need only pharmacotherapy to improve do not lose time in and incur the expense of psychotherapy. If there is an inadequate response to antidepressants alone or to a change in medication, psychotherapy is then added. Psychotherapy must usually be combined with pharmacotherapy in patients with multiple symptom clusters that might respond differentially to psychotherapy, as well as in patients with severe or chronic depression. However, it may be necessary to produce at least some improvement in energy, motivation, and cognition with a medication before the patient can participate meaningfully in psychotherapy.

Because addition of IPT to antidepressants reduced the attrition rate from 21% to 8% in the continuation therapy study involving patients with recurrent unipolar depression (Frank et al. 1990), psychotherapy should be included in the maintenance treatment of recurrent unipolar depression, even if the index episode was not severe. However, adding psychotherapy to antidepressants may be more efficient than starting both treatments at the same time, unless barriers to compliance with drug therapy are identified at the start of treatment or the mood disorder is more severe or complex.

Certain problems frequently complicate decisions about combining psychotherapy and pharmacotherapy. Some therapists who assume that depression is caused by repressed emotions begin treatment by encouraging patients to attempt to remember events that must be linked with depression. Patients who have experienced loss and trauma may believe that it is necessary to express grief and feelings about being traumatized if depression is to be cured. Although it may be very useful to address these issues once depression has been adequately treated, depression may intensify further strong dysphoric emotions and conflicts, making it impossible to deal with them. Failure to resolve these issues and eliminate depression makes the patient feel like more of a failure, which further intensifies depression.

Although no psychotherapy has been shown to be effective by itself for either pole of bipolar disorder, this modality is often necessary to address noncompliance and to help stabilize circadian rhythms. IPSRT and reduction of expressed emotion in the family can also improve mood in bipolar disorder. In addition, many people with bipolar mood disorders have developed psychological and social complications of an unstable mood that may be integrated into their views of themselves and their interactions with others. Important targets for exploratory psychotherapy include problematic behaviors such as driving people away before they have a chance to leave, stimulus seeking, or getting into situations that evoke strong emotions—all of these behaviors being engaged in to create the illusion of being in control of mood swings that are really unpredictable. Once the mood disorder is under better control, attention can be directed toward ways in which the patient's personality has been built around a chronically unstable mood.

Even though they have not been tested as primary treatments for mood disorders, conjoint and family therapy should be added to somatic therapies whenever possible. Assortative mating and familial transmission of mood disorders result in an increased familial prevalence of these conditions. Family members may encourage or interfere with treatment compliance, and family stress is intensified by an active mood disorder in a family member. When patients do not respond as expected, it is especially important to evaluate contributing factors in the family.

■ REFERENCES

Agency for Health Care Policy and Services Research: Clinical Practice Guidelines: Depression in Primary Care, Vol 2: Treatment of Major Depression. Rockville, MD, U.S. Department of Health and Human Services, 1993

Blackburn I-M, Eunson KM, Bishop S: A two-year naturalistic follow-up of depressed patients treated with cognitive therapy, pharmacotherapy, and a combination of both. J Affect Disord 10:67–75, 1986

Brown RA, Lewinsohn PM: A psychoeducational approach to the treatment of depression: comparison of group, individual, and minimal contact procedures. J Consult Clin Psychol 52 (5):774–783, 1984

Budman SH, Deniby A, Redondo JP, et al: Comparative outcome in time-limited individual and group psychotherapy. International Journal of Group Psychotherapy 38:63–86, 1998

Crits-Christoph P: The efficacy of brief dynamic psychotherapy: a meta-analysis. Am J Psychiatry 149 (2):151–158, 1992

Elkin I, Shea MT, Watkins JT, et al: National Institute of Mental Health Treatment of Depression Collaborative Research Program: general effectiveness of treatments. Arch Gen Psychiatry 46:971–982, 1989

Evans MD, Hollon SD, DeRubeis RJ, et al: Differential relapse following cognitive therapy and pharmacotherapy for depression. Arch Gen Psychiatry 49:802–808, 1992

Flint AJ, Rifat SL: The effect of sequential antidepressant treatment on geriatric depression. J Affect Disord 36 (3–4):95–105, 1996

Frank E, Kupfer DJ, Perel JM, et al: Three-year outcomes for maintenance therapies in recurrent depression. Arch Gen Psychiatry 47:1093–1099, 1990

Frank E, Kupfer DJ, Wagner EF, et al: Efficacy of interpersonal psychotherapy as a maintenance treatment of recurrent depression: contributing factors. Arch Gen Psychiatry 48:1053–1059, 1991

Frank E, Hlastala S, Ritenour A, et al: Inducing lifestyle regularity in recovering bipolar disorder patients: results from the maintenance therapies in bipolar disorder protocol. Biol Psychiatry 41:1165–1173, 1997

Gabbard GO: Psychodynamic psychotherapies, in Treatments of Psychiatric Disorders, 2nd Edition. Edited by Gabbard GO. Washington, DC, American Psychiatric Press, 1995, pp 1205–1220

Gallagher-Thompson D, Hanley-Peterson P, Thompson LW: Maintenance of gains versus relapse following brief psychotherapy for depression. J Consult Clin Psychol 58:371–374, 1990

Herson M, Bellack AS, Himmelhoch JM, et al: Effects of social skills training, amitriptyline, and psychotherapy in unipolar depressed women. Behavior Therapy 15:21–40, 1984

Hollon SD, Fawcett J: Combined medication and psychotherapy, in Treatments of Psychiatric Disorders, 2nd Edition. Edited by Gabbard GO. Washington, DC, American Psychiatric Press, 1995, pp 1221–1236

Hollon SD, DeRubeis RJ, Evans MD, et al: Cognitive therapy and pharmacotherapy for depression: singly and in combination. Arch Gen Psychiatry 49:774–781, 1992

Jarrett RB: Comparing and Combining Short-Term Psychotherapy and Pharmacotherapy for Depression. New York, Guilford, 1997

Katon W, Rutter C, Ludman EJ, et al: A randomized trial of relapse prevention of depression in primary care. Arch Gen Psychiatry 58:241–247, 2001

Keller MB, McCullough JP, Klein DN, et al: A comparison of nefazodone, the cognitive behavioral-analysis system of psychotherapy, and their combination for the treatment of chronic depression. N Engl J Med 342:1462–1470, 2000

Kupfer DJ, Frank E, Perel JM: Five-year outcome for maintenance therapies in recurrent depression. Arch Gen Psychiatry 49:769–773, 1992

McLean PD, Hakstian AR: Relative endurance of unipolar depression treatment effects: longitudinal follow-up. J Consult Clin Psychol 58 (4):482–488, 1990

Meterissian GB, Bradwejn J: Comparative studies on the efficacy of psychotherapy, pharmacotherapy, and their combination in depression: was adequate pharmacotherapy provided? J Clin Psychopharmacol 9 (5):334–339, 1989

Miklowitz DJ, Simoneau TL, George EL, et al: Family focused treatment of bipolar disorder: 1-year effects of a psychoeducational program in conjunction with pharmacotherapy. Biol Psychiatry 8:582–592, 2000

Reynolds CF 3rd, Frank E, Perel JM, et al: Maintenance therapies for late-life recurrent major depression: research and review circa 1995. Int Psychogeriatr 7 (suppl):27–39, 1995

Roose SP, Stern RH: Medication use in training cases: a survey. J Am Psychoanal Assoc 43:163–170, 1995

Roth D, Bielsky R, Jones M, et al: A comparison of self-control therapy and combined self-control therapy and antidepressant medication in the treatment of depression. Behavior Therapy 13:133–144, 1982

Stuart S, Thase ME: Inpatient application of cognitive behavior therapy: a review of recent developments. J Psychother Pract Res 3:284–299, 1994

Thase ME: Long-term treatments of recurrent depressive disorders. J Clin Psychiatry 53 (suppl):32–44, 1992

Thase ME: Reeducative psychotherapies, in Treatments of Psychiatric Disorders, 2nd Edition. Edited by Gabbard GO. Washington, DC, American Psychiatric Press, 1995, pp 1169–1204

Thase ME, Kupfer DJ: Recent developments in the pharmacotherapy of mood disorders. J Consult Clin Psychol 64:646–659, 1996

Thase ME, Greenhouse JB, Frank E, et al: Treatment of major depression with psychotherapy or psychotherapy-pharmacotherapy combinations. Arch Gen Psychiatry 54:1009–1015, 1997

Wilson PH: Combined pharmacological and behavioural treatment of depression. Behav Res Ther 20 (2):173–184, 1982

6

INTEGRATED TREATMENT OF UNIPOLAR DEPRESSION

The "Practice Guideline for Major Depressive Disorder in Adults" (American Psychiatric Association 1993) states that successful treatment of mood disorders begins with a careful diagnostic, psychosocial, and medical evaluation along with consideration of the patient's treatment preferences. The initial assessment of a patient with a mood disorder (and all subsequent treatment) occurs in the context of a relationship between doctor and patient. This interaction is crucial to the development of a therapeutic alliance in which the patient collaborates with the physician. In the National Institute of Mental Health Treatment of Depression Collaborative Research Program, the therapeutic alliance significantly affected outcomes of interpersonal psychotherapy, cognitive-behavioral therapy, active pharmacotherapy, and administration of placebo (Blatt et al. 1996). Treatment dropout rates are less than 10% when a collaborative alliance has been fostered (Frank et al. 1995).

Informed consent is an essential component of a therapeutic alliance. Because no treatment is clearly established as superior to other reasonable therapies for most mood disorders, the process of obtaining consent should involve a discussion of alternative therapies, the evidence in favor of and against the treatment course that is being recommended, and the likely outcome of no treatment. This approach might mean informing a patient that a course of psychotherapy being suggested has not been proven to be effective for depression but has been useful in the therapist's experience. The same statement can be made about the many pharmacological regimens for refractory mood disorders that have not been tested in controlled trials. Psychosis and mania do not necessarily make informed consent impossible, but severely depressed patients may feel so hopeless that they do not believe that anything will help, whereas manic patients may believe that nothing is the matter with them.

Evaluation of risk factors for suicide (see Introduction) is essential in all patients with mood disorders. Because suicidal patients (especially those with psychotic mood disorders, bipolar illness, or both) may kill someone else before they kill themselves, homicide risk should also be evaluated. The risk of infanticide should be evaluated in women with postpartum psychosis. Dangerousness is not a static issue but one that evolves with the mood disorder. It is therefore necessary to reevaluate dangerousness to self and others repeatedly throughout the treatment of a mood disorder. It is also important to inquire about nonsuicidal forms of self-destructive behavior, which are particularly common in patients with comorbid mood and personality disorders and also occur in some patients with bipolar mood disorders.

Review of the patient's use of substances that can cause or aggravate depression or mania (Table 1–15) is another essential component of the evaluation of a patient with a mood disorder. Active depression may inhibit abstinence from substances, and concomitant treatment of depression and substance use may be necessary (see Chapter 1). However, it is much more difficult to treat a mood disorder in a patient who is actively using alcohol or illicit drugs. Because the presence of comorbid disorders such as medical illness, panic disorder, eating disorders, obsessive-compulsive disorder, generalized anxiety, social phobia, posttraumatic stress disorder, or personality disorders can alter prognosis and call for a modification of the treatment, it is also important to diagnose these disorders in patients with mood disorders.

The next important step is to decide whether the mood disorder is unipolar or bipolar. Such a distinction is crucial, given the different treatment approaches to the two disorders. When a patient has a clear-cut history of mania, the diagnosis is straightforward. However, bipolar disorder may be more difficult to identify when a patient has had one or a few depressive episodes without obvious manic or hypomanic symptoms. Clues to bipolarity in a depressed patient are summarized in Table 6–1, although like all other aspects of mood disorders, the bipolar–unipolar distinction is one that may be clarified only with continued observation.

TABLE 6–1.   **Clues to bipolarity in depressed patients**

Highly recurrent depression
Intense anger
Racing thoughts
Mood-incongruent psychotic symptoms
Hallucinations
Thrill seeking
Increased libido with severe depression
Family history of bipolar disorder
Three consecutive generations with mood disorders

■ MAJOR DEPRESSIVE DISORDER

A mildly or moderately severe single major depressive episode without psychotic features can be treated with antidepressants or psychotherapy. However, the longer the duration of the episode, or the greater its severity, the more likely an antidepressant is to be needed. Even if formal psychotherapy is not provided, antidepressant prescriptions should at least be accompanied by informed psychological management that maximizes the therapeutic alliance and helps the patient voice concerns about the treatment and bring up issues that may complicate treatment. Because the presence of a comorbid personality disorder or perfectionism predicts a poorer response to antidepressants as well as to briefer psychotherapies, more intensive forms of psychodynamic psychotherapy may be appropriately added to treatment with antidepressants when these factors are present, although empirical support for this approach has not yet emerged. Conjoint therapy should be considered for patients with more complicated depression, because interpersonal issues are often important to address and because depressed patients often have relatives who are depressed. In view of the fact that treatment of depression in a primary care setting is much less likely to include psychotherapy in any form than is treatment by mental health professionals, which produces better results, more efforts should be made to include competent psychotherapy in the treatment of depressed primary care patients.

Although all antidepressants currently available are equally effective, all antidepressants are not equally effective for all patients. Perhaps because of differences in drug disposition and receptor responsiveness, many patients who do not respond to one agent will respond to another. The initial choice of an antidepressant generally depends on the patient's history and current symptoms. For example, patients who have had good responses to a particular antidepressant may respond to the same medication again, although an antidepressant that was effective at one point may not work as well when it is readministered after having been discontinued. Insomnia associated with depression often improves with remission of depression, but more sedating antidepressants such as doxepin, imipramine, trazodone, mirtazapine, and nefazodone can produce more rapid relief of insomnia, whereas more activating antidepressants such as fluoxetine, bupropion, and tranylcypromine can aggravate insomnia. Because of their marked antihistaminic properties, trimipramine and doxepin can be useful for treating allergies and peptic ulcer disease, and nefazodone may be useful for treating fibromyalgia.

Despite the role of serotonin in pain, selective serotonin reuptake inhibitors (SSRIs) have not proven as useful for chronic pain as tricyclic antidepressants (TCAs) and nefazodone. Mirtazapine and venlafaxine may have potential for treating chronic pain, and substance P antagonists would theoretically be useful for comorbid depression and chronic pain. Conversely, SSRIs and bupropion are safer than TCAs in patients with heart block and possibly in patients with recent myocardial infarctions. Patients who experience nausea with cancer chemotherapy and those with significant weight loss or insomnia respond well to mirtazapine, the chewable preparation of which is useful for older patients who have difficulty swallowing pills. Patients with atypical depression appear to respond most frequently to monoamine oxidase inhibitors (MAOIs) and least frequently to TCAs (which are still more effective than placebo); SSRIs are intermediate in efficacy (Quitkin et al. 1991).

Because major depression is associated with high levels of physiological arousal as well as hypervigilance for negative events, depressed patients are often hypersensitive to medication side effects. Although patients with milder and more acute forms of depression may tolerate rapid dose escalation, very slow adjustment of the antidepressant dose often improves tolerability of the drug, especially in patients who are anxious and therefore in a higher state of arousal. Having the patient contact the physician after each dose increase reduces the patient's anxiety about the medication and provides an opportunity to encourage the patient to continue treatment. If the dose of an antidepressant is kept below the threshold for intolerable side effects, tolerance often develops and the dose can be gradually increased. Conversely, if adverse effects are initially more severe, tolerance is less likely to develop, making it much more difficult to achieve a therapeutic dose.

Antidepressant overdose is the most common method of suicide in the United States. A large body of clinical experience contradicts a report of a small number of cases in which suicidal ideation was thought to be increased by SSRIs and indicates that the risk of suicide is reduced by all antidepressants—including SSRIs, which decrease inwardly as well as outwardly directed impulsive aggression (Isacsson et al. 1996). Because newer antidepressants are safer in overdose than TCAs, the best initial choices for suicidal patients may be SSRIs, venlafaxine, mirtazapine, and nefazodone. Prescribing small quantities of antidepressants to a suicidal patient in an attempt to prevent the patient from taking a lethal overdose forces the patient to make frequent trips to the pharmacy, which may encourage noncompliance and indirectly increase the risk of suicide because depression is undertreated. If the risk of suicide is so great that the physician cannot trust the patient with an antidepressant, the patient should be hospitalized.

Once recovery with antidepressant therapy begins, its time course is the same as spontaneous remission, suggesting that antidepressants may speed recovery but not change its natural course. One implication of this finding is that treatment with antidepressants should be continued acutely for at least as long as the depressive episode would be expected to last if it remained untreated. Achieving a complete remission may take longer than the 4–6 weeks traditionally recommended for acute treatment of major depression. For example, in a cohort of 56 patients with major depressive disorder (MDD) treated with pharmacotherapy and psychotherapy, 49% of patients had full remissions, and 45% had partial remissions, after 9 months (Van Londen et al. 1998). Over the next 3–5 years of continued treatment, 82% had full remissions; 16% of patients required 2 years to achieve full remission. During the same period, 41% of the sample had recurrences. Similarly, when a group of patients with chronic major or double depression who had partially responded after 3 months of treatment with an SSRI or a TCA were randomized to continued treatment with the same medication (Miller and Freilicher 1995), 50% had remissions, and 30% had partial responses, over the next 4 months. Although such findings do not support continuation of treatment with ineffective antidepressants for extended periods, they may be an indication that patients responding slowly to an antidepressant may simply have a slower course of recovery.

Debate continues about which antidepressant is best for severe depression. Well-publicized controlled studies found clomipramine to be superior to the SSRIs citalopram and paroxetine in severely depressed inpatients (Danish University Antidepressant Group 1986, 1990). However, not all controlled studies support the hypothesis that TCAs are more effective than SSRIs in more severe forms of unipolar depression (Nierenberg 1994). This issue remains unresolved because detecting a statistically significant difference in the efficacy of two active antidepressants requires the inclusion of more than 350 patients in each treatment group and in the placebo group and is otherwise methodologically difficult. Electroconvulsive therapy (ECT) is a particularly appropriate option for patients who are too severely depressed or suicidal to wait for an antidepressant to take effect, patients who cannot tolerate an antidepressant, and patients with associated illnesses that might benefit from ECT, such as delirium or Parkinson's disease.

A substantial amount of information has accumulated about the treatment of major depression with psychotic features. Psychotic depression has a very low rate of spontaneous recovery and responds virtually not at all to placebo or psychotherapy alone (Dubovsky and Thomas 1992). Only 0%–46% (average, about 25%–35%) of patients with psychotic depression respond to TCAs; MAOIs do not produce better results. Whereas 19%–48% of psychotically depressed patients recover with the use of neuroleptic medications alone, the combination of a neuroleptic and an antidepressant leads to improvement in an average of 70%–80% of patients (Dubovsky and Thomas 1992; Spiker et al. 1986). It is not known whether mild or transient psychotic symptoms convey the same treatment requirements as more pervasive or severe psychosis.

Combination therapy involves more than differential treatment of psychosis by the antipsychotic drug and depression by the antidepressant, because neuroleptic therapy alone ameliorates depression in some patients and antidepressant therapy alone ameliorates psychosis in others (Dubovsky and Thomas 1992). Higher neuroleptic doses than those used for schizophrenia may be needed for psychotic depression (Spiker et al. 1986). Amoxapine, an antidepressant that is a metabolite of the neuroleptic loxapine and that has neuroleptic properties of its own, is almost as effective as traditional neuroleptic–antidepressant combinations in psychotic depression (Anton and Burch 1986). The primary drawbacks of this treatment are that neuroleptic and antidepressant doses cannot be adjusted separately and the neuroleptic cannot be withdrawn, which means that the patient is subjected to the ongoing risk of tardive dyskinesia. The rate of response of psychotic depression is greatest with ECT. As discussed in Chapter 4, combinations of antidepressants and neuroleptic drugs may be effective for severe nonpsychotic depression.

The antidepressant properties of atypical antipsychotic agents, and their lower risk of neurological side effects, make these medications appealing choices for psychotic depression. Rothschild et al. (1999) reviewed records of 15 hospitalized patients with discharge diagnoses of unipolar or bipolar depression with psychotic features who were treated with olanzapine. Comparing these records with those of matched patients who took antipsychotics (most patients in each treatment group were also taking antidepressants), the investigators found a higher rate of improvement among patients treated with olanzapine. Preliminary experience suggests that atypical antipsychotic drugs may also be effective as single agents in psychotic depression (McElroy et al. 1991). Obviously, controlled prospective trials would be necessary to determine whether atypical antipsychotic drugs may be effective alone or in combination with antidepressants.

In the office treatment of psychotic unipolar depression, the initial treatment depends on the severity and nature of the patient's symptoms. A patient with severe agitation or psychosis might be given an antipsychotic drug first, and an antidepressant might be added once the patient was less agitated. A patient with milder psychosis could be treated initially with an antidepressant, and the antipsychotic drug might be added if all symptoms did not remit completely with the antidepressant alone. Patients with pervasive psychosis and severe depression should probably begin combination therapy.

Because the risk of bipolarity is increased in younger patients with psychotic depression, especially those with hallucinations without delusions, these patients should be evaluated for features listed in Table 1–16. The treatment of psychotic bipolar depression is discussed in Chapter 7.

The goal of remission rather than only response is often not achieved with a single antidepressant (or with medications without psychotherapy), especially in patients with more severe or chronic depression. Because residual symptoms increase the risk of relapse and recurrence, it is important to treat these vigorously. The clinician can begin by asking questions listed in Table 6–2. When these issues and psychosocial and family issues have been addressed, deciding whether to augment or change the antidepressant is a matter of clinical judgment. Experience suggests that antidepressants should be changed if they have had no positive effect at all after at least 4–6 weeks at therapeutic doses, as should medications that are poorly tolerated at low doses, whereas augmentation is more successful when the patient has had a partial response. Of the agents that have been used to augment antidepressants in unipolar depression (Table 6–3), lithium has been the best studied. Augmentation with buspirone and gabapentin may be most useful for anxious depression. Triiodothyronine augmentation may be most effective in the presence of subclinical hypothyroidism. Stimulant augmentation seems most useful for older patients. Whereas tolerance develops to the antidepressant effect of these medications when used as single agents, this has not been as much of a problem when stimulants are used for augmentation of antidepressants. Stimulants and modafinil can also be used to treat sedation caused by antidepressants, as well as to augment treatment with them. Augmentation of antidepressants with antipsychotic drugs may be effective for refractory nonpsychotic depression.

When deciding whether to make antidepressant therapy more aggressive, it is important to distinguish between nonclinical drops in mood and covert residual symptoms since only the latter increase the risk of relapse. One differentiating point is that symptoms suggesting partial relapse are similar to those of the previous episode and tend to worsen over time, whereas nonclinical mood swings are primarily stress related and do not resemble symptoms of previous depressive episodes. When actual evidence of relapse exists, psychosocial issues should be addressed before the antidepressant regimen is changed, because patients respond with the same symptoms to losses, helplessness, unexpressed anger, and related states as they do to the endogenous physiology of depression.

After initial improvement, response to an antidepressant sometimes fades. A review of published double-blind, placebo-controlled trials with at least 20 patients reporting loss of antidepressant efficacy during maintenance treatment found this problem to be present

---

TABLE 6–2. **Questions for evaluating inadequate antidepressant response**

Are the dose and duration of treatment adequate?

Is the patient taking the medication?

Is a medical illness contributing to treatment resistance?

Is the patient taking a medication or substance that is interfering with the antidepressant?

Is the patient truly depressed?

Are psychotic symptoms present?

Is the depression bipolar?

Are psychosocial issues being ignored?

Has the patient's family been involved in treatment?

TABLE 6–3. **Agents used to augment antidepressant therapy in unipolar depression**

Lithium

Stimulants

Carbamazepine

Buspirone

T_3

Gabapentin

Atypical antipsychotic drugs

SSRI–TCA combination

Mirtrazapine–venlafaxine combination

MAOI–TCA combination

Note. MAOI=monoamine oxidase inhibitor; SSRI=selective serotonin reuptake inhibitor; TCA=tricyclic antidepressant; T_3=triiodothyronine.

in 9%–33% of patients (Byrne and Rothschild 1998). Relapse during the first 12 weeks was believed to reflect loss of an initial placebo response, especially when features of a placebo response such as abrupt, fluctuating improvement were present initially. The authors found 75 cases that were thought to demonstrate tolerance to antidepressants after full remission rather than loss of a placebo effect. Tolerance to antidepressants has been reported with serotonin reuptake inhibitors, heterocyclic antidepressants, and MAOIs.

There are a number of possible mechanisms of tolerance to anti-depressants. A common problem with antidepressants that induce their own metabolism or are taken along with other medications (such as carbamazepine) that induce metabolizing enzymes is pharmacokinetic tolerance or a decrease in serum levels to below the therapeutic range. This problem is usually corrected with one or more increases in dose until levels remain constant. Pharmacodynamic tolerance is probably caused by intracellular mechanisms that attempt to restore the premorbid "default" state by overriding the response of receptors or intracellular targets to the medication. In this situation, increasing the dose of an antidepressant may produce a brief return of therapeutic benefit, but this wears off rapidly and a change in medication or a medication combination is likely to be necessary. Treatment with fluoxetine is sometimes associated with the late development of a therapeutic window, possibly owing to accumulation of a long-acting metabolite, levels of which may be negatively correlated with antidepressant efficacy of the parent drug. This problem necessitates a reduction rather than an increase in the dose of the antidepressant.

Certain varieties of treatment-emergent loss of antidepressant benefit require a more global reconsideration of the pharmacological strategy. The most important of these is bipolar depression masquerading as recurrent or fluctuating unipolar depression. The antidepressant is effective initially, but because it accelerates the tendency of bipolar depression to recur as well as its tendency to remit, another episode appears that is mistaken for loss of antidepressant efficacy. A change in the antidepressant produces another remission, but this is inevitably followed by another recurrence, often mixed with dysphoric hypomanic symptoms such as anxiety, intense irritability, racing thoughts, the inability to shut one's mind off and get to sleep, severe interpersonal sensitivity, or subtle psychotic symptoms. Whereas continuing to change the dose or preparation of the antidepressant produces more recurrences and sometimes more persistent depression, adding a mood-stabilizing medication and gradually withdrawing the antidepressant often eliminates depressive recurrences. Management of bipolar depression is discussed at greater length in Chapter 7.

It is commonly recommended that patients continue taking an effective antidepressant for 4–12 months after remission of a single major depressive episode. However, this recommendation is based only on observational data and a small number of discontinuation studies. In the National Institute of Mental Health Collaborative Study of the Psychobiology of Depression, 359 patients treated for a unipolar major depressive episode who decided themselves whether to continue taking an antidepressant were reexamined every 6 months for 2 years and every year for another 3 years. Among patients with less recurrent depression, the risk of recurrence was highest during the first 8 months and then decreased to a weekly rate of 1%, which suggests that the benefit of continuing the use of an antidepressant decreased after 8 months of continuation treatment. However, the recommendation for an 8-month continuation phase may be overly optimistic, given that patients who elected to stop taking antidepressants may have been aware of having a less severe and recurrent condition. In fact, most patients did not have severe or recurrent depression, and patients in the study who had five previous episodes had many more recurrences after withdrawal of antidepressants. In other studies, elderly patients with major depression were significantly less likely to have a recurrence while taking antidepressants for 8 months to 2 years. The conventional wisdom that maintenance doses of antidepressants can be lower than therapeutic doses was contradicted by several studies comparing relapse and recurrence rates at therapeutic and half-therapeutic antidepressant doses (Frank et al. 1993).

It is usually suggested that an antidepressant be discontinued as slowly as possible, because withdrawal of an antidepressant over weeks to months seems to be associated with a reduced risk of recurrence of major depression. In addition to a theoretically reduced risk of rebound and recurrence, this approach makes it easier to reinstitute treatment before the medication has been completely withdrawn. Very slow withdrawal of medication also reduces discontinuation syndromes, which are common with shorter-acting antidepressants such as paroxetine and venlafaxine, even when the sustained-release formulation of the latter is used. However, there are no controlled comparisons of slow versus rapid tapering of antidepressant doses.

Given the current state of knowledge, the most conservative recommendation is that treatment with an effective antidepressant be continued for at least 8 months after remission of a single episode of unipolar depression that did not produce severe impairment or suicidality, and then that the antidepressant be withdrawn over 2–4 months. Patients who have had three or more episodes should probably take an antidepressant—one that has been effective acutely—indefinitely. Patients with a single recurrence after many years of feeling well might reasonably opt to discontinue an antidepressant again, whereas those with a recurrence soon after an index episode should continue treatment. Among patients who have had a single severe or life-threatening episode, the risk of a recurrence is probably greater than the risk and inconvenience of continuing treatment with the antidepressant.

In view of evidence that continuation psychotherapy treats residual symptoms and psychosocial dysfunction that predispose to relapse, psychotherapy that has proven useful should probably also be continued at some frequency under the same circumstances that antidepressant therapy would be continued. Continued contact with a clinician also facilitates monitoring for relapse. However, aside from an older finding that when combined with imipramine, monthly interpersonal psychotherapy further reduced relapse risk (Kupfer et al. 1992), there are few data on the optimal "dose" of maintenance psychotherapy.

An interesting approach to the question of how long to continue psychotherapy after a single depressive episode was applied in a comparison of two studies involving patients with MDD who responded to cognitive therapy (CT) (Jarrett et al. 1998). In study 1, treatment was discontinued after an acute response in 37 patients, who were then followed prospectively for 24 months. In the second 2-year study, 17 patients with MDD who responded acutely to CT received 8 months of continuation CT. Treatment was then stopped, and patients were followed without treatment for another 16 months. Recurrence rates in study 1 were 40% at 6 months, 50% at

12 months, and 74% at 24 months. In study 2, recurrence rates were 20% at 6 months, 27% at 12 months, and 36% at 24 months after acute treatment. The findings suggested that the additional 8 months of continuation CT produced lower recurrence rates over a total of 2 years of follow-up. In actual practice, patients with recurrent major depression would continue psychotherapy at an optimal frequency indefinitely.

■ DYSTHYMIC DISORDER AND CHRONIC MAJOR DEPRESSION

Placebo-controlled trials demonstrate that dysthymia responds as well as major depression does to TCAs, SSRIs, MAOIs, and atypical antidepressants such as tianeptine, although rates of noncompliance related to demoralization and intolerance of adverse effects are high. In a comparison of the effect of ECT in 25 patients with double depression and 75 patients with episodic MDD, Prudic et al. (1993) found that both groups demonstrated the same level of improvement in depression rating-scale scores. However, patients with double depression had more residual symptoms and were more likely to relapse in the year after ECT, which suggests that the underlying dysthymia was incompletely treated.

Psychotherapies that have been found useful for treating chronic depressive disorders include CT, interpersonal psychotherapy, behavior therapy, cognitive-behavioral therapy, supportive therapy, psychoeducation, and family and marital therapy (Akiskal 1994). However, the response to psychotherapy is less robust than in acute depression. Combining structured psychotherapies with antidepressants produces better results than medication therapy alone in dysthymic patients (Frances 1993). Maintenance pharmacotherapy as well as psychotherapy is particularly important for reducing the risk of recurrence of dysthymia, and of chronic major depression and double depression. As is true of major depressive episodes, the more complete the treatment, the lower the risk of relapse and recurrence.

■ RECURRENT BRIEF DEPRESSION

Only a few studies of the treatment of recurrent brief depression have been conducted. Obviously, there would not be enough time for an antidepressant to produce remission of acute episodes lasting less than 2 weeks. However, antidepressants do not appear to be nearly as effective in preventing depressive recurrences as in treating recurrent MDD. Lithium may reduce recurrences, even though no evidence has emerged of a bipolar outcome in recurrent brief depression (Angst and Hochstrasser 1994). It is not known whether other mood-stabilizing medications might reduce the rate of recurrence of this form of depression, but given that these medications have antirecurrence as well as antimanic properties, it seems reasonable to consider using them for this action. If recurrent brief depression is considered a mood disorder in which a bipolar trait (i.e., a high rate of recurrence) is combined with a depression that is unipolar in form, the possibility must be considered that chronic use of antidepressants could have the potential to speed up the rate of recurrence of acute depressive episodes. This hypothesis awaits formal testing.

■ SEASONAL AFFECTIVE DISORDER

The use of artificial bright light in the treatment of seasonal affective disorder (SAD) is discussed in Chapter 4. Most commercial bright lights now have intensities of 10,000 lux, and patients treated with such lights usually require just 30 minutes of exposure per day. Ongoing bright light therapy is necessary to prevent relapse, which often occurs within 3–5 days of discontinuing the light therapy. Winter recurrences can be prevented by initiating bright light therapy when days begin to get shorter (usually September to early November in the Northern Hemisphere) and continuing it until days begin to get longer (late March to late April).

A number of medications, including fluoxetine, moclobemide, tranylcypromine, bupropion, and alprazolam, have been observed to be at least as effective as bright light for treating SAD. Whereas some patients prefer bright light because it is not a medication and has no real interactions, others find antidepressants more convenient, especially if they travel frequently. In the case of patients with yearly recurrences of seasonal depression, prophylactic bright light therapy is usually begun in the early fall and continued through the spring. Some clinicians use seasonal administration of antidepressants for the same purpose, but this approach has not been formally compared to maintenance treatment with an antidepressant or a mood stabilizer. Patients with bipolar SAD can be treated with seasonal use of bright light or a thymoleptic or both, depending on response to the light and whether thymoleptics alone prevent seasonal recurrences.

Artificial bright light can also be used as an adjunct to antidepressants in the treatment of major depression with winter exacerbation. This treatment is particularly useful for patients with hypersomnia or a phase delay of their sleep–wake cycle. Exposure to light in the morning helps correct this problem by phase-advancing the sleep–wake cycle, which helps the patient feel more alert during the day. The best "dose" of bright light can be determined by gradually increasing the duration of exposure until the patient responds.

■ UNIPOLAR DEPRESSION IN CHILDREN AND ADOLESCENTS

Experience with antidepressants has not been as positive in younger patients as it has been in adults. In placebo-controlled trials, the efficacy of TCAs has consistently been found to be equivalent to the efficacy of placebo in children and inferior to the efficacy of placebo in adolescents with major depression (Geller et al. 1996). There are several possible explanations for these findings. The rates of placebo response and spontaneous improvement may be so high in depressed juvenile patients that it is impossible to demonstrate a differential effect of active treatment. Environmental factors, especially those related to the family, have more influence on treatment response in some younger patients, and unless these are addressed, antidepressants may be less effective. Fear of giving medications to children in the first place and lack of knowledge about the tendency of younger patients to eliminate medications more rapidly than older patients may result in inadequate dosing. Once-daily dosing, which is effective with many antidepressants in adults, may produce serum levels that are not as consistent in children and younger adolescents. In some cases, early-onset depression may be more severe and therefore more likely to be refractory to treatment. High rates of bipolarity and comorbidity could also contribute to lower rates of response to antidepressants in younger patients, whose illnesses may be biologically different from adult mood disorders. Finally, not all results of antidepressant trials involving adults have been positive, and there may not have been a sufficient number of controlled trials involving children and adolescents to yield consistently positive results.

Childhood and adolescent depression is often accompanied by atypical features, and it has been suggested that treatment with MAOIs may be more effective than treatment with TCAs, but dietary noncompliance is often a problem with MAOI therapy. SSRIs are safer and better tolerated in younger populations. One of two controlled studies of fluoxetine in children and adolescents demonstrated superiority of fluoxetine to placebo, and one study showed no difference between placebo and active drug (Geller et al. 1996). A controlled study of venlafaxine in 33 patients ages 8–17 years showed no differences between active drug and placebo, but doses were very low, and patients given placebo as well as those given venlafaxine also received psychotherapy (Mandoki et al. 1997). Fluoxetine, sertraline, paroxetine, fluvoxamine, and venlafaxine have been found effective in trials of varying rigor in children and adolescents and appear to be more effective than TCAs. ECT is about as effective and safe in juvenile patients as it is in adults (Walter and Rey 1997), but obtaining informed consent is more difficult, and fears of the treatment are greater.

Children and adolescents should be treated first with individual and/or family psychotherapy; more intensive psychotherapies may be more likely to produce full recovery (Geller et al. 1996). Patients who do not respond to psychotherapy might be given an SSRI before any other class of antidepressant. The high rate of bipolar outcome and the lack of prospective studies of antidepressant maintenance therapy warrant discontinuation of antidepressants at some point after remission, but the timing of this intervention remains to be studied.

■ MAINTENANCE TREATMENT OF UNIPOLAR DEPRESSION

As was discussed in "Major Depressive Disorder," the recommendation that antidepressants be continued for 4–12 months after a single episode of unipolar major depression is based only on observational data and a few discontinuation studies and does not take into account the ability of antidepressants to prevent recurrence (50% of patients not treated with antidepressant maintenance therapy experience recurrence within 2 years of remission of a first episode [Consensus Development Panel 1985]). The decision to withdraw an antidepressant after the first major depressive episode is therefore more complex than it might appear at first. Obviously, patient preference is a crucial factor. Depressed patients often do not like taking antidepressants for extended periods. Cost and adverse effects are considerations, but many patients object even more to the idea of needing a medication, because this need signifies that the patient is weak, dependent, or ill.

Even acutely, between 33% and 68% of depressed patients have been found to be noncompliant with antidepressant therapy, and the rate of long-term treatment adherence is even lower (Burrows 1992). More than 20% of patients do not fill the first antidepressant prescription, and most patients who do begin treatment stop medications within 14 weeks. Patients who are reluctant to accept help may insist on the lowest possible dose of an antidepressant, as if this were equivalent to the lowest possible amount of assistance. Ease of use (i.e., less-frequent dosing) and a lower incidence of adverse effects explain why the likelihood of filling a third prescription for an SSRI is twice that of filling a third prescription for a TCA, despite the greater cost of the SSRI.

The clinical importance of nonadherence was illustrated in a prospective review of Medicaid records of 4,052 adult patients who received a prescription for a TCA or an SSRI at the time of receiving a diagnosis of depression (Melfi et al. 1998). During the 2-year follow-up, 70% of patients filled fewer than four prescriptions, and only 19% used antidepressants continuously. Discontinuation of an antidepressant was associated with a 77% increase in the risk of relapse or recurrence, whereas the likelihood of relapse or recurrence was lowest among patients who continued taking antidepressants.

The risk–benefit ratio of continuing antidepressant therapy is another factor to consider when deciding whether to continue treatment with an antidepressant after a first major depressive episode. If the episode was relatively mild and easy to treat, the risk of discontinuing antidepressants is relatively low. Conversely, if the episode was severe or had major consequences such as a serious suicide attempt, an inability to work, or disruption of the family, the risk of another episode may be substantially greater than the inconvenience of continuing antidepressant treatment. If depression responded only after multiple antidepressant trials, the benefit of continuing antidepressant therapy may outweigh the risk of another long and difficult course of treatment if depression recurs. After improvement of depression with psychotherapy or pharmacotherapy, relapse and recurrence are up to five times more likely to occur after treatment withdrawal if residual symptoms are present (Thase et al. 1992). Slower antidepressant withdrawal may be less likely to be followed by rebound and relapse than rapid drug discontinuation. However, no controlled comparisons of slow versus rapid tapering of antidepressant doses have been done.

There have been no extended studies of antidepressant discontinuation after treatment of a first or second major depressive episode. However, after three or more episodes, withdrawal of an antidepressant has been found to be associated with an increased risk of recurrence for at least 5 years after remission (Kupfer et al.

1992). In view of reliable data indicating that relapse and recurrence of unipolar depression are reduced by continuation of antidepressant therapy (Fava and Kaji 1994), patients with recurrent unipolar depression should continue to take an effective antidepressant indefinitely. Of 23 prospective, double-blind, randomized studies of continuation and maintenance pharmacotherapy for depression, 22 found more recurrences in the placebo group, and the only study that detected no difference involved too few patients to be reliable (Solomon and Bauer 1993). The same dose that produced remission appears necessary to prevent recurrence (Blackburn 1994; Devanand et al. 1991; Frank et al. 1993).

Since 1987, at least 25 reports on the use of continuation or maintenance ECT have suggested that such therapy can decrease rehospitalization rates by two-thirds or more (Petrides et al. 1994). Continuation or maintenance ECT is frequently administered on an outpatient basis, which increases patient acceptance. The frequency of maintenance treatments is based on symptom emergence as the time between ECT treatments is gradually increased. Because medications that were ineffective before ECT are no more effective after successful ECT, maintenance ECT for an indefinite period is often recommended after remission.

Refilling prescriptions or prescribing other maintenance somatic therapies without at least intermittently reviewing treatment adherence and residual or prodromal symptoms increases the risk that nonadherence and relapse will be missed until the patient is grossly symptomatic. Because cognitive therapy (CT), cognitive-behavioral therapy, and interpersonal psychotherapy, when combined with antidepressants, have been shown to further reduce the risk of recurrence of unipolar depression and to treat residual symptoms that have not remitted with antidepressant therapy, there is good reason to assume that continuation, possibly at a reduced frequency, of one of these psychotherapies—or any other psychotherapeutic approach that has proven useful in acute depression—along with the antidepressant will reduce the risk of relapse or recurrence of major depression or dysthymia (Fava and Kaji 1994; Kupfer et al. 1992; Weissman 1994).

In a study by Jarrett et al. (2001), patients who achieved remission of an acute episode of unipolar depression with a standard course of CT (20 sessions) were randomly assigned to either no continuation CT or 10 sessions of continuation CT over a period of 8 months. Sixteen months after the conclusion of the continuation phase, the risk of relapse and recurrence was significantly reduced in the group that received continuation CT. This finding may suggest that the benefit of maintenance psychotherapy persists longer than the benefit of maintenance pharmacotherapy after treatment discontinuation. An alternative explanation is that the relatively prolonged benefit of a continuation phase of psychotherapy was due to the study patients' being less severely ill than patients in studies of maintenance pharmacotherapy. Another possible explanation is that recurrences began after the follow-up period. In actual practice, a single course of psychotherapy may produce a remission that persists as long as or even longer than a spontaneous remission; however, without some form of maintenance therapy, recurrences are likely, especially in patients who have already had depressive recurrences.

The recommendation that psychotherapy be continued after remission of depression is not easy to implement in an era of cost containment that limits visits to a clinician after a patient is well. However, the cost of maintenance psychotherapy may be much less than the cost of treating another major episode, which could prove more difficult to treat than to prevent, especially if there is any residual psychosocial dysfunction. Patients who prefer to avoid the perception of needing help unless they are desperate or who must pay for treatment out of pocket may be especially likely not to continue treatment once they feel well. In the latter phase of psychotherapy, attention might be directed toward assessing the real risk of relapse, the chance that maintenance treatment will reduce that risk, and the ability of the family to at least develop a plan for monitoring the patient for early return of symptoms that might indicate the need for a follow-up appointment.

Residual dysfunction commonly persists after remission of specific depressive symptoms. In addition to attenuated depressive symptoms, residual symptoms may include personality problems, social maladjustment, interpersonal friction, inhibited communication, poor work or school performance, and dysfunctional attitudes. Patients often overlook subsyndromal residual symptoms, and physicians may mistake them for indications of a comorbid personality disorder. It is not uncommon for patients and their physicians to discontinue treatment at this point, with important consequences. Over time, patients experience deterioration of self-esteem, an increase in dysfunctional attitudes, greater functional and role impairment, an increase in the use of medical services, and increases in suicide risk and the risk of recurrence and relapse. Partially recovered depressed patients with Hamilton Rating Scale for Depression scores in the range of 8–14 (who in most antidepressant studies would be considered as having responded to treatment) have a 25%–45% probability of objective work impairment and a 60%–80% probability of subjective work impairment and are more likely not to respond to further treatment. Like patients with residual depressive symptoms, patients with residual social dysfunction are at high risk for relapse and recurrence. Conversely, patients who are completely asymptomatic are less likely to have recurrences than those with residual symptoms.

One reason residual symptoms increase the risk of relapse and recurrence may be that they indicate that the pathophysiology of depression has not yet resolved. Another marker of residual pathophysiology of depression, indicating incomplete remission, is persistence of biological markers such as dexamethasone nonsuppression (as determined by the dexamethasone suppression test) or electroencephalographic sleep changes, both of which predict a greater risk of relapse or recurrence. Residual symptoms may also represent symptoms that were present before the acute episode but were initially overshadowed by more florid acute symptoms and were not eliminated by acute treatment (see Chapter 3). Such symptoms then become prodromes of a new episode.

Preventing the negative effect of residual symptoms on current functioning and later likelihood of recurrence involves several principles. The finding that as many as 46% of patients with partial remissions ultimately achieved full remission with continuation of aggressive treatment is an indication for continuing acute treatment for a longer period in chronically depressed patients if improvement has not reached a distinct plateau at a level lower than remission. However, it is important to use the most aggressive treatment possible, including augmentation strategies, so that a remission rather than just a response is produced. As discussed in Chapter 5, use of psychotherapy to treat residual psychological symptoms such as negative cognitions reduces the risk of recurrence after drug discontinuation, so the addition of psychotherapy to pharmacotherapy is usually indicated for patients who have had incomplete remissions with pharmacotherapy alone.

■ APPROACHES TO MANAGED CARE

Recommendations for combined antidepressant therapy and psychotherapy, aggressive treatment of residual symptoms, indefinite maintenance schedules with regular checkups for patients who have recovered from recurrent major depression, and prescriptions for more than a month's supply of medication at a time are usually inconsistent with managed care protocols, the goals of which involve discontinuation of everything but medication after alleviation of an acute episode, as well as frequent requests for approval by a case manager of any kind of physician– or therapist–patient contact. Although such protocols may make sense for patients with a single episode of major depression of mild to moderate severity without associated complicated psychosocial pathology, it is more cost-effective to apply appropriate maintenance strategies than to keep treating recurrences, which may become more complex and refractory. While the insurance company may save money in the short term by withholding approval for aggressive maintenance therapy, the cost to society of further recurrences and residual symptoms outweighs the cost of initial care.

A proactive approach to the conflict between formulas directed by the short-term bottom line and the patient's need for a longer-term strategy may be more successful than reacting to treatment denials at a time when the patient may be ambivalent about the maintenance phase anyway. Because acute treatment of chronic or recurrent major depression is only the first phase of a prolonged intervention, case managers should be involved early in long-term planning, and appeals mechanisms should be explored early in treatment. When the patient and the family are prepared in advance for the possibility that they will have to be active in dealing with inappropriate attempts to limit ongoing treatment, they become more involved in the overall treatment process. Appeals and reports to the National Committee for Quality Assurance, which certifies most managed care organizations, may convince managed care reviewers to certify chronic treatment after initial refusals, but these actions, as well as complaints to the benefits offices of employers, must be initiated by patients and their families, who must have at least the hope that their efforts will be successful.

■ REFERENCES

Akiskal HS: Dysthymic and cyclothymic depressions: therapeutic considerations. J Clin Psychiatry 55:46–52, 1994

American Psychiatric Association: Practice guideline for major depressive disorder in adults. Am J Psychiatry 150:1–26, 1993

Angst J, Hochstrasser B: Recurrent brief depression: the Zurich Study. J Clin Psychiatry 55 (suppl):3–9, 1994

Anton RF, Burch EA: Amoxapine versus amitriptyline combined with perphenazine in the treatment of psychotic depression. Am J Psychiatry 147:1203–1208, 1986

Blatt SJ, Sanislow CA 3rd, Zuroff DC, et al: Characteristics of effective therapists: further analyses of data from the National Institute of Mental Health Treatment of Depression Collaborative Research Program. J Consult Clin Psychol 64:1276–1284, 1996

Burrows GD: Long-term clinical management of depressive disorders. J Clin Psychiatry 53 (suppl):32–35, 1992

Byrne SE, Rothschild AJ: Loss of antidepressant efficacy during maintenance therapy: possible mechanisms and treatments. J Clin Psychiatry 59:279–288, 1998

Consensus Development Panel: NIMH/NIH Consensus Development Conference statement. Mood disorders: pharmacologic prevention of recurrences. Am J Psychiatry 142:469–476, 1985

Danish University Antidepressant Group: Citalopram: clinical effect profile in comparison with clomipramine: a controlled multicenter study. Psychopharmacology (Berl) 90:131–138, 1986

Danish University Antidepressant Group: Paroxetine: a selective serotonin reuptake inhibitor showing better tolerance, but weaker antidepressant effect than clomipramine in a controlled multicenter study. J Affect Disord 18:289–299, 1990

Dubovsky SL, Thomas M: Psychotic depression: advances in conceptualization and treatment. Hospital and Community Psychiatry 43:1189–1198, 1992

Fava M, Kaji J: Continuation and maintenance treatments of major depressive disorders. Psychiatric Annals 24:281–290, 1994

Frances AJ: An introduction to dysthymia. Psychiatric Annals 23:607–608, 1993

Frank E, Kupfer DJ, Perel JM, et al: Comparison of full-dose versus half-dose pharmacotherapy in the maintenance treatment of recurrent depression. J Affect Disord 27:139–145, 1993

Frank E, Kupfer DJ, Siegel LR: Alliance not compliance: a philosophy of outpatient care. J Clin Psychiatry 56 (suppl 1):11–16, 1995

Geller B, Todd RD, Luby J, et al: Treatment-resistant depression in children and adolescents. Psychiatr Clin North Am 19:253–265, 1996

Isacsson G, Bergman U, Rich CL: Epidemiological data suggest antidepressants reduce suicide risk among depressives. J Affect Disord 41:1–8, 1996

Jarrett RB, Basco MR, Risser R, et al: Is there a role for continuation phase cognitive therapy for depressed outpatients? J Consult Clin Psychol 66:1036–1040, 1998

Jarrett RB, Kraft D, Doyle J, et al: Preventing recurrent depression using cognitive therapy with and without a continuation phase: a randomized clinical trial. Arch Gen Psychiatry 58:381–388, 2001

Kupfer DJ, Frank E, Perel JM: Five-year outcome for maintenance therapies in recurrent depression. Arch Gen Psychiatry 49:769–773, 1992

Mandoki MW, Tapia MR, Tapia MA, et al: Venlafaxine in the treatment of children and adolescents with major depression. Psychopharmacol Bull 33:149–154, 1997

McElroy SL, Dessain EC, Pope HG Jr, et al: Clozapine in the treatment of psychotic mood disorders, schizoaffective disorder, and schizophrenia. J Clin Psychiatry 52:411–414, 1991

Melfi CA, Chawla AJ, Croghan TW, et al: The effects of adherence to anti-depressant treatment guidelines on relapse and recurrence of depression. Arch Gen Psychiatry 55:1126–1132, 1998

Miller FT, Freilicher J: Comparison of TCAs and SSRIs in the treatment of major depression in hospitalized geriatric patients. J Geriatr Psychiatry Neurol 8 (3):173–176, 1995

Nierenberg AA: The treatment of severe depression: is there an efficacy gap between SSRI and TCA antidepressant generations? J Clin Psychiatry 55 (suppl A):55–59, 1994

Petrides G, Dhossche D, Fink M, et al: Continuation ECT: relapse prevention in affective disorders. Convulsive Therapy 10:189–194, 1994

Prudic J, Sackeim HA, Devanand DP, et al: The efficacy of ECT in double depression. Depression 1:38–44, 1993

Quitkin FM, Harrison W, Stewart JW, et al: Response to phenelzine and imipramine in placebo nonresponders with atypical depression: a new application of the crossover design. Arch Gen Psychiatry 48:319–323, 1991

Rothschild AJ, Bates KS, Boehringer KL, et al: Olanzapine response in psychotic depression. J Clin Psychiatry 60:116–118, 1999

Solomon DA, Bauer MS: Continuation and maintenance pharmacotherapy for unipolar and bipolar mood disorders. Psychiatr Clin North Am 16:515–540, 1993

Spiker DG, Perel JM, Hanin I, et al: The pharmacological treatment of delusional depression: part II. J Clin Psychopharmacol 6:339–342, 1986

Thase ME: Reeducative psychotherapies, in Treatments of Psychiatric Disorders. Edited by Gabbard GO. Washington, DC, American Psychiatric Press, 1995, pp 1169–1204

Thase ME, Simons AD, McGeary J, et al: Relapse after cognitive behavior therapy of depression: potential implications for longer courses of treatment. Am J Psychiatry 149:1046–1052, 1992

Van Londen L, Molenaar RPG, Goekoop JG, et al: Three- to 5-year prospective follow-up of outcome in major depression. Psychol Med 28:731–735, 1998

Walter G, Rey J: An epidemiological study of the use of ECT in adolescents. J Am Acad Child Adolesc Psychiatry 36:809–815, 1997

Weissman MM: Psychotherapy in the maintenance treatment of depression. Br J Psychiatry 165 (suppl 26):42–50, 1994

7

INTEGRATED TREATMENT OF BIPOLAR DISORDER

Although there are important differences between the treatment of unipolar and bipolar mood disorders, in both groups of conditions it is necessary to consider the longitudinal course of the illness when treating any acute episode. An expert consensus panel that compiled opinions of 58 national experts agreed that mood-stabilizing medications should be used in all phases of treatment of bipolar disorder (Sachs et al. 2000). The consensus panel suggested lithium or divalproex as the initial agent, with carbamazepine as the next choice. Antipsychotic medications were recommended for psychotic bipolar disorder and as adjuncts for severe nonpsychotic mania and mixed states. Anticonvulsants were preferred over lithium for mixed states and rapid cycling.

■ MOOD CHARTS

Treatment of bipolar disorder is complicated by unpredictable fluctuations in mood, different treatment protocols for mixed states, and state-dependent recall. The latter phenomenon makes it difficult for patients to remember accurately how they felt when they were in one mood state and experiencing different affects. For example, a patient who feels depressed in the clinician's office may not recall having felt energized or even elated the previous day. Patients with very rapid mood swings may simply not be able to keep track of their numerous complicated affective experiences. Antidepressants are less effective during ultradian (ultrarapid) cycling and mixed states. A prospective mood chart is therefore useful, because it can help clinician and patient decide which treatment to introduce at which point.

Post et al. (1988) and others (Roy-Byrne et al. 1985) developed a life-charting method that quantifies symptoms and important life events. However, life charting is time-consuming and relies on observations by nursing staff. In everyday outpatient practice, it may be equally helpful to construct with the patient a graph on which specific symptoms are rated one or more times per day using whatever scale makes the most sense (e.g., mood can be rated from –5 [very depressed] to +5 [manic], with 0 signifying euthymia). Different symptoms such as depressed mood, irritability, racing thoughts, suicidal ideation, self-destructive behavior, and increased or decreased sleep can be indicated by different line colors or styles, and changes in treatment as well as important events can be noted on the same graph. However it is accomplished, prospective mood charting can be essential in tracking mixtures of depressive, hypomanic, and psychotic symptoms to determine whether to add more mood-stabilizing medications, an antipsychotic drug, or an antidepressant or to withdraw a particular treatment. Graphic ratings are usually easier to evaluate than narrative comments. Patients who are skillful with spreadsheets may prefer to enter numerical scores and print them as a graph. One example of a simple mood chart is presented in Figure 7–1.

■ MANIA

Lithium, carbamazepine, and valproic acid (divalproex) appear to be equally effective in the treatment of acute mania; response rates range from 40% to 70% (American Psychiatric Association 1994). Lithium is the best studied and most clearly established of these agents; verapamil has not been subjected to multicenter studies, although smaller studies suggest it is most useful for mania that is responsive to lithium. Treatment with lithium may be less effective than treatment with anticonvulsants in mixed (dysphoric) and psychotic mania (McElroy et al. 1992). Treatment with combinations

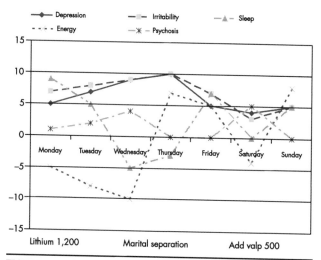

FIGURE 7–1. **Sample mood chart.**

of antimanic drugs may be more effective than treatment with a single medication. Like all affective episodes, mania should be viewed in the context of the longitudinal course of the illness, and the need for immediate control of symptoms should be balanced against the need to maximize long-term acceptability of the treatment.

Activated states in bipolar disorder have a number of typical presentations, ranging from frank mania to hyperthymia (Table 7–1). Points to be covered in the initial evaluation of the manic patient are summarized in Table 7–2, and beginning-treatment strategies are outlined in Figure 7–2. Although patients with mild forms of mania and supportive families may be managed in outpatient or partial care settings, more severely agitated, assaultive, or self-destructive patients usually must be hospitalized. Because the onset of action of most antimanic drugs is not immediate, antipsychotic drugs and/ or benzodiazepines can be used to treat psychosis, reduce aggressive behavior, and enhance sleep (enhancing sleep often improves mania).

246

TABLE 7–1.   Presentations of mania

Pure mania
Psychotic mania
Mixed mania
Delirious mania
Postpartum psychosis
Hypomania
Hyperthymia

TABLE 7–2.   Points to cover in the initial evaluation of the manic patient

Suicide or homicide risk
Impulsivity
Assaultiveness
Substance use
Presence of mixed and psychotic symptoms
Number of previous episodes
Previous course
Treatments effective or ineffective in the past
Compliance history
Degree of social disruption, and available supports
Medical illnesses

The first step with any patient is to ensure the safety of patient and staff. Group meetings, discussions of emotionally loaded material, and other interactions should generally be minimized at first, because manic patients are easily overstimulated. At the same time that they are less overwhelmed if they can be physically isolated from the milieu, manic patients are often driven toward contact with others in an attempt to regulate unstable affective systems. Seclusion may be necessary for patients who become dangerously overstimulated in any interaction but cannot isolate themselves. Even though many patients are aware that they are likely to feel better if they are by themselves, they experience a pressure for interaction that makes it very difficult to withdraw from interpersonal contact. As a result, some seclusions may have to involve sufficient staff to contain the patient safely.

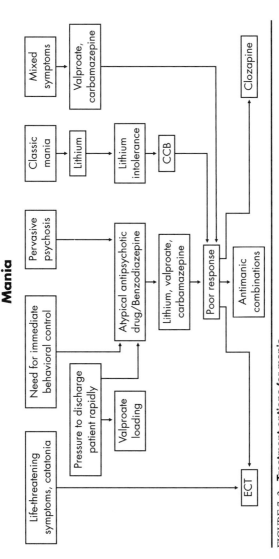

FIGURE 7–2. **Treatment options for mania.**

Abbreviations: CCB=calcium-channel blocker; ECT=electroconvulsive therapy.

It takes longer to control behavioral and affective dysregulation in mania than is usually mandated in managed care protocols; therefore, many manic patients are "outliers." To reduce the risk of premature discharge of the patient, it is helpful to contact the managed care reviewer in advance to discuss the treatment protocol. Discharging a patient to the community before affective systems are sufficiently stabilized may result in rapid relapse as the patient becomes overstimulated.

The choice of initial antimanic treatment depends on the urgency of the situation (Figure 7–2). If behavioral control is not immediately necessary, treatment with an antimanic drug can be initiated. Pure mania (i.e., nonpsychotic mania that is not mixed with depression) may respond equally to lithium, an anticonvulsant, or a calcium channel–blocking agent. The latter agents, especially verapamil, are most useful for patients who responded to lithium but could not tolerate it, patients with concomitant dementia, and pregnant patients with mania. However, calcium-channel blockers are not usually effective as single agents in refractory or mixed mania. Most experts recommend initiating treatment for dysphoric mania with divalproex or carbamazepine.

Rapid oral loading of divalproex and aggressive use of antipsychotic medications can help to reduce acute manic symptoms quickly, which is particularly useful when patients are dangerously agitated or near exhaustion, or when sufficient resources to contain the patient are not available. However, this approach can interfere with long-term treatment. Adverse effects, which may not be apparent until drug accumulation occurs after discharge, may lead the patient to discontinue treatment. Rapid escalation of antimanic doses may also be more likely than slower escalation to eliminate mania before eliminating mixed depression that has been obscured by mania, and the patient will be left feeling more acutely lethargic or depressed and be more likely to withdraw from therapy. One way to avoid this problem is to use benzodiazepines and/or antipsychotic drugs for agitation and insomnia and gradually increase the dose of a mood-stabilizing medication as the initial drug or drugs are gradually withdrawn. For hospitalized patients, the antimanic drug dose can gradually be increased after discharge, and medications for insomnia and agitation can be slowly withdrawn.

Until recently, neuroleptics (particularly haloperidol) were used routinely to control agitation until the antimanic drug took effect. However, not all manic patients are psychotic, and psychosis accompanying mania may remit with adequate treatment of the mania. Supplementation of neuroleptic therapy with the benzodiazepines lorazepam or clonazepam was introduced as a means of minimizing neuroleptic exposure with its attendant risks of side effects and adverse interactions with antimanic drugs.

Because atypical antipsychotic drugs seem to be equally effective for psychotic and nonpsychotic mania (Tohen et al. 2000), atypical antipsychotics can be used with or without benzodiazepines to treat acute mania, but given the current state of knowledge, they should be considered supplements to treatment with established antimanic drugs since their mood-stabilizing properties (i.e., their ability to reduce affective recurrences) have not been proven. Once the patient's behavior is under better control, an attempt should be made to withdraw antipsychotic medications as an antimanic drug is gradually introduced. Although some patients, especially those with persistent severe depression, may benefit from continuation of treatment with an atypical antipsychotic medication, the possibility that antidepressant actions of these medicines may eventually predominate should be kept in mind. Electroconvulsive therapy (ECT) is the most rapidly effective treatment for the affective as well as the behavioral manifestations of mania.

■ BIPOLAR DEPRESSION

There have been fewer controlled studies of the treatment of bipolar depression than of other forms of depression. However, American Psychiatric Association practice guidelines for the treatment of bipolar disorder (American Psychiatric Association 1994), the Expert Consensus Guidelines (Sachs et al. 2000), and some investigators (Compton and Nemeroff 2000) recommend, in view of the risk of antidepressant-induced mania and rapid cycling (see Chapter 3), that treatment of bipolar depression begin with an antimanic drug. This approach is illustrated in Figure 7–2. Lithium has been noted to be an effective antidepressant in 30%–79% of patients with bipolar depression; its antidepressant efficacy is comparable to the efficacy of antidepressants (Zornberg and Pope 1993). The finding that a full response to lithium took up to 8 weeks in nine controlled studies (Zornberg and Pope 1993) may imply that the treatment trial was inadequate in studies with a lower response rate. Carbamazepine was better than placebo in three of three controlled studies of bipolar depression (Zornberg and Pope 1993). Divalproex can be effective for depressive symptoms occurring during a manic episode and for more subtle mixed states, but it is often not very effective as a primary antidepressant in patients without mixed hypomanic symptoms. Lamotrigine has more obvious antidepressant properties (Sachs et al. 2000), but because it may not be as effective against manic recurrences as it is against depressive recurrences, it is probably safer to combine it with a well-established antimanic drug.

When bipolar depression does not remit with administration of an antimanic drug, the clinician must decide whether to add a second antimanic drug or an antidepressant. Antimanic drugs are not as effective as antidepressants for treating depression and have more adverse effects, but all antidepressants carry the risk of inducing mania and rapid cycling. In the absence of controlled data, only clinical experience and expert opinion guide the choice between these two courses. Experience suggests that antidepressants do not produce a predictably positive response in bipolar depression with prominent mixed hypomanic symptoms such as profound irritability, decreased sleep without tiredness during the day, racing thoughts, extreme interpersonal sensitivity, hallucinations, or increased libido. Instead, antidepressants provoke more dysphoric hypomania or produce initial improvement followed by more recurrences of mixed bipolar depression. Treatment with a combination of antimanic drugs may produce a remission or may at least convert a refractory mixed state to a less complicated bipolar depression with hypersomnia, lethargy, slowed thinking, and lack of interpersonal sensitivity—a depression that may respond more predictably to the addition of an antidepressant (Figure 7–3).

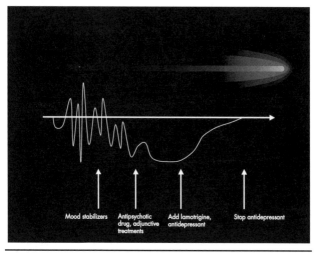

FIGURE 7–3. **Treatment of bipolar depression.**

The combination of lithium and carbamazepine has been found to have antidepressant properties in some studies (Post 1988). Verapamil has been used to treat bipolar depression in a few cases, but it is usually not effective as an antidepressant; of the calcium-channel blockers, nimodipine seems more useful for bipolar depression as well as for brief recurrent depression. Lamotrigine can be an effective antidepressant, and preliminary studies suggest that it can at least reduce the number of recurrences of bipolar depression and possibly hypomania (Calabrese et al. 1999, 2001). Antipsychotic drugs may be necessary adjunctively when psychotic symptoms complicate manic symptoms mixed with depression, but if used too long, antipsychotics may aggravate depression, and newer atypical antipsychotic medications can have unpredictable effects. Clozapine appears to have distinct mood-stabilizing properties that can be useful in complex mixed bipolar depression to eliminate at least the dysphoric hypomanic component (Zarate et al. 1995).

Although it is often possible to eliminate mixed dysphoric hypomania with combinations of mood stabilizers, they are often not effective acutely for depression. When this lack of effectiveness becomes apparent, an antidepressant must be added. It seems clear that antidepressants should normally not be administered to patients with bipolar depression unless an antimanic drug is coadministered (Sachs et al. 2000). However, the choice of a specific antidepressant in treating bipolar depression is limited by lack of replicated data. Given accumulating data supporting lamotrigine's antidepressant action in bipolar depression, this drug is an appropriate first choice for patients who can tolerate it. The fact that the dose must be increased slowly (12.5–25 mg/week) to minimize the risk of a severe rash may not be a problem for some patients, because the antidepressant effect of this medication may not be apparent at lower doses.

Another early treatment for depression, especially winter bipolar depression, is artificial bright light. An important advantage of bright light is that the dose can be adjusted very precisely. It may be possible to find a duration of exposure that treats depression without inducing hypomania. Stimulants are generally not used as primary antidepressants in unipolar depression because tolerance to their antidepressant action develops over several months, but the rapid onset and short duration of stimulants' antidepressant effect can be useful in treating bipolar depression. As is true of bright light, the rapid onset of action helps produce a prompt antidepressant response, and the rapid offset of action can be beneficial if hypomania or cycling develops during treatment.

If these interventions are not effective, one of the more traditional antidepressants is added. Tricyclic antidepressants are generally thought to be more likely than bupropion, monoamine oxidase inhibitors (MAOIs), and selective serotonin inhibitors (SSRIs) to induce mania and rapid cycling. However, this impression may come from findings of some earlier studies of antidepressants in unipolar depression, studies in which investigators were not as accurate in excluding patients with bipolar disorder as other investigators have been in studies of newer antidepressants.

Nevertheless, many experts recommend that bupropion or an SSRI be given as an initial antidepressant and that venlafaxine or tranylcypromine be used for refractory bipolar depression (Thase and Sachs 2000). The greatest amount of empirical data are available for tranylcypromine in bipolar depression (Nolen and Bloemkolk 2000). Dietary restrictions associated with MAOI use are obviously troublesome, but the duration of antidepressant treatment may not be long enough to make these restrictions intolerable.

A number of alternatives or supplements to antidepressants can be considered in treating bipolar depression that does not respond to combinations of mood stabilizers and antidepressants. Atypical antipsychotic drugs other than clozapine have antidepressant properties that can be useful in severe nonpsychotic as well as psychotic bipolar depression. As discussed in Chapter 4, pramipexole has been effective in a few patients with refractory bipolar depression. In several controlled studies of bipolar depression, ECT was superior to antidepressants (Zornberg and Pope 1993). Unlike other antidepressant therapies, ECT rarely induces mania, and when it does, further ECT usually normalizes mood.

There is no evidence that continuation of treatment with antidepressants after remission of bipolar depression prevents further depressive recurrences (Loo and Brochier 1995). In view of the risks of long-term antidepressant therapy, it seems prudent to attempt to withdraw the antidepressant once mood normalizes, while continuing the mood-stabilizing regimen (Sachs et al. 2000). Gradual discontinuation of antidepressants (over months) may reduce the risk of rebound depression, which can lead to the mistaken impression that the antidepressant is still needed. If it becomes necessary to continue treatment with the antidepressant, lower doses may be less likely to destabilize mood, but mood stabilizers may prove to be more effective at preventing recurrences of depression than they are at treating depression acutely, whereas continuing the antidepressant for too long may result in cycling into more depression. Maintenance ECT can prevent recurrences of bipolar depression as well as recurrences of mania.

■ MIXED AND RAPID-CYCLING BIPOLAR DISORDER

Rapid cycling is the most common diagnosis in patients with refractory bipolar disorder. Although the response rate of uncomplicated mania to lithium in three relatively recent trials ranged from 59% to 91%, response rates among patients with mixed states and rapid cycling were only 29%–43% (Gershon and Soares 1997). Rapid cycling and mixed states are generally thought to have a lower response to lithium than more sustained affective episodes and perhaps a greater rate of response to divalproex or carbamazepine (Kusumakar et al. 1997). However, when carbamazepine and lithium were directly compared in patients with rapid-cycling bipolar disorder, both drugs were found to be equally effective (Okuma 1993). A consensus panel recommended valproate as the first choice for treating rapid cycling; carbamazepine and lithium were the recommended second and third choices, respectively (Expert Consensus Panel for Bipolar Disorder 1996).

Despite the substantial heterogeneity of rapid-cycling variants of bipolar disorder, an overall approach similar to the treatment of bipolar depression (Figure 7–3) can be useful. It is important (even more important than it is in the treatment of mania) to view the primary complaint at the moment in the context of the longitudinal course of bipolar disorder. Directing treatment immediately toward one pole of the mood disorder, especially depression, is less effective than first addressing the problem of recurrence. It is helpful to remember that even though patients with rapid and especially ultradian cycling are usually in a good deal of distress, they have been ill for quite some time. Clinical experience demonstrates that responding to the patient's sense of urgency, especially with regard to relief of depression, often results in longer treatment trials. Rapid escalation of the dose of any medication does not give the patient time to become tolerant to side effects and may result in noncompliance. In addition, when the dose of a mood-stabilizing medication is increased too quickly, the medication is more likely to act initially against mixed dysphoric hypomania than against depression. In such cases, symptoms such as irritability, anxiety, insomnia, and agitation remit, but patients experience more of the very depression they were trying to treat.

Because most patients with rapid cycling are depressed when they enter treatment (Calabrese et al. 2001), they are usually taking antidepressants or demand immediate treatment with these agents. Such patients find it much more difficult to tolerate depression than to tolerate hypomania (even if the latter is extremely dysphoric) because they prefer feeling activated to feeling anergic. However, the first step in treating rapid cycling is to withdraw antidepressants slowly and focus on treatment with mood stabilizers, at least until cycling and mixed dysphoric hypomania remit. A mood chart will help the clinician determine prospectively when both cycling and mixed symptoms such as irritability and insomnia have been completely treated. Consensus guidelines discussed at the beginning of the chapter recommend divalproex as the first agent; the next choices recommended are lithium, other anticonvulsants, and possibly nimodipine. Case series suggest that combinations of two or three mood stabilizers may be more effective than a single agent in the treatment of rapid cycling (Post et al. 2000), which is no different than the treatment of any refractory medical illness in which multiple medications with different mechanisms of action are necessary to address multiple dysregulated cellular processes.

As we noted in Chapter 4, preliminary research suggests that lamotrigine may be especially useful for bipolar depression (Calabrese et al. 2000; Walden et al. 2000). In a study apparently involving some of the same patients described by Calabrese et al. (2000), patients with refractory bipolar disorder were treated openly for 48 weeks with lamotrigine, either as an adjunctive ($n=60$) or single ($n=15$) agent (Bowden et al. 1999). The majority (71%) of rapid-cycling patients did not complete the entire study. Using the last observation carried forward, it was found that patients with rapid cycling demonstrated significant symptomatic and functional improvement, but rapid-cycling patients had less improvement of mania than non-rapid-cycling patients. The finding that depression improved more than mania suggests that lamotrigine may be more useful for patients with bipolar disorder who are predominantly depressed.

As we described in Chapter 4, nimodipine may be a useful third-line treatment for rapid cycling in patients who cannot tolerate or do not respond to other treatments. In our experience with nimodipine, it has appeared to be more effective for refractory bipolar illness when it is combined with other mood stabilizers than as monotherapy. Adverse reactions with carbamazepine are less likely than they are with verapamil, and nimodipine may be more useful than verapamil when depression predominates.

The use of antipsychotic medications in rapid cycling is similar to the use of these medications in bipolar depression. The threshold for using antipsychotic drugs for intractable mood cycling and psychosis is usually lower than when psychosis is not present, but antipsychotic drugs can also be helpful in reducing mood cycling in refractory nonpsychotic rapid cycling. Clozapine is probably most reliably effective for this purpose. Newer atypical antipsychotic medications are sometimes helpful, especially when patients complain primarily of depression, but at times the antidepressant action of these medications, especially at higher doses, can aggravate rapid cycling. Neuroleptics other than loxapine do not generally have significant antidepressant properties, although they can contribute to depression once cycling is eliminated. Lower doses of antipsychotic drugs are often preferable for rapid cycling.

Correction of subclinical hypothyroidism, which is present in as many as 70% of patients with rapid cycling, may make this condition more responsive to treatment. Replacement therapy may produce better results when given as 75% T_4 and 25% T_3, with the aim of normalizing thyroid function. It was noted as early as the 1930s (Gjessing 1938) that high doses of thyroid hormone have a positive effect on cyclical mood disorders. As a result, supraphysiological doses of thyroid hormone have been used adjunctively in patients with rapid cycling as summarized in Chapter 4. Risks of this treatment and the small body of data supporting it make use of suprametabolic doses of thyroid to treat rapid cycling, or other bipolar presentations appropriate only if no other treatments were helping.

Altering the timing of sleep and awakening with adjunctive use of artificial bright light in the morning may be helpful in treating rapid cycling (see Chapter 4). Enforced sleep using a prolonged lights-out protocol, combined with morning bright light, may stabilize the sleep–wake cycle and help normalize mood in rapid cycling. Morning bright light without enforced sleep has also been used to stabilize the sleep–wake cycle and treat depression in patients with refractory rapid cycling (Kusumi et al. 1995).

If cycling is slowly reduced with carefully adjusted combinations of mood stabilizers, possibly supplemented with antipsychotic drugs or, in more drastic cases, thyroid medication, cholinesterase inhibitors, acetazolamide, choline, tamoxifen, or other experimental therapies mentioned in Chapter 4, the patient's mood may gradually normalize. However, it seems more common in clinical practice for mood to stabilize in a low state in which more-classic bipolar depression persists, with anergia, hypersomnia, slowed thinking, and related symptoms but without significant fluctuation of mood, extreme interpersonal sensitivity, or mixed hypomanic symptoms. In one of the few studies of this issue, a combination of lithium and divalproex administered openly for 6 months to patients with rapid cycling prevented mania in 85% and depression in 60%; only 50% of patients had prevention of both mania and depression (Calabrese et al. 2001). In some cases, treatment-emergent depression will cycle away on its own, and mood stabilizers will gradually attenuate recurrences. However, for patients with more persistent depression, the challenge of finding an antidepressant regimen that will not restore cycle acceleration is the same as the challenge of finding the most effective antidepressants for the treatment of bipolar depression (Figure 7–4).

Lithium–carbamazepine combinations might be considered for treatment of rapid cycling as well as for treatment of bipolar depression. Although valproate is probably less likely to treat depression successfully, it may prevent cycling into another depressive episode as soon as the first one remits. If depression persists, lamotrigine may be a good initial choice because its mood-stabilizing effect is more reliable in the presence of depression than of mania. For

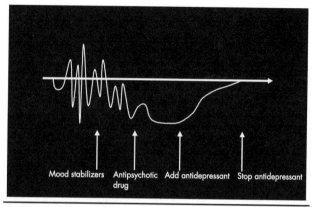

FIGURE 7–4. **Mood chart.**

patients with a phase delay in the sleep–wake cycle, morning bright light can help both normalize sleep and relieve depression; the duration of exposure must be titrated carefully. Stimulants, SSRIs, bupropion, and MAOIs are subsequent choices, as they are in the treatment of bipolar depression. An activating atypical antipsychotic medication might also be considered.

How long to continue treatment with antidepressants after remission of depression in patients with rapid cycling is a question that remains controversial. The opinion that continuing antidepressant therapy for too long may induce more mood cycling has been criticized as unnecessarily stringent, given the existence of antidepressants that might be less likely to have this effect (Moller and Grunze 2000). However, the majority of experts still recommend withdrawing antidepressants after depression remits (Sachs et al. 2000); slow withdrawal of the antidepressant reduces the risk of rebound depression. If relapse appears anyway, the antidepressant might be reintroduced and then withdrawn once the depression remits again.

For patients who cannot tolerate or do not respond to medications, ECT can be effective in eliminating rapid cycling. For example, a patient who developed rapid cycling after starting treatment with an antidepressant and who did not respond to thymoleptic combinations achieved a complete remission with six ECT treatments (Berman and Wolpert 1987). In open trials of ECT in 20 patients who had mixed affective disorders that did not respond to treatment with lithium and/or carbamazepine, 3 of 8 patients with rapid cycling had ECT-induced remissions lasting 5 months or more (Mosolov and Moshchevitin 1990). Findings of an open trial of ECT in 6 patients who had continuous cycling suggested that affective recurrences were more likely to be diminished when cycling started within a few months of institution of ECT than when ECT was begun later in the course of rapid cycling (Wolpert et al. 1999). Such observations in keeping with clinical experience suggesting that ECT, like other treatments, is not as effective in treating established rapid cycling as might be predicted, especially when the illness does not respond to other treatments. In addition, patients with rapid cycling who do respond to ECT may need a large number of treatments. Because many patients with rapid cycling are treated with multiple agents, a greater possibility of interactions with ECT exists.

■ MAINTENANCE TREATMENT OF BIPOLAR DISORDER

The high rates of affective recurrence, as well as the increasing abruptness, severity, and complexity of each recurrence, are reasons to continue a mood-stabilizing regimen after remission of any acute episode of mania or bipolar depression. A mood chart is especially helpful in maintenance therapy.

At least 10 double-blind, placebo-controlled studies, each involving more than 200 patients, have demonstrated that lithium substantially reduces the number of manic and depressive recurrences: in these studies, 0%–44% of patients taking lithium had recurrences, compared with 38%–93% of patients taking placebo (Solomon and Bauer 1993). Recurrence rates were reduced by an average of 50% (range, 21%–97%) in 11 studies involving 877 patients (Davis et al. 1999). Serum lithium levels greater than 0.8 mEq/L are associated with significantly lower recurrence rates than levels less than 0.6–0.8 mEq/L, but adverse effects are more common at higher levels (Davis et al. 1999). The prophylactic effect of lithium results in a substantial decrease in suicide rates, and this decrease results in the addition of 7 years to life expectancy. In a study involving 405 patients with bipolar mood disorders and 92 patients with unipolar depression, all treated in a lithium clinic, the suicide rate increased by 80% if patients left the clinic and discontinued lithium, and the rate increased by 45% if patients left the clinic but continued to take lithium (Kallner et al. 2000).

Carbamazepine therapy was effective as a maintenance treatment in bipolar illness in four published trials; however, lack of a placebo control in three of these trials, and only a trend toward superiority of carbamazepine in the one placebo-controlled trial, limits the strength of this conclusion (Solomon et al. 1995). Maintenance treatment with carbamazepine was as effective as lithium maintenance therapy, over 1–3 years, in 10 studies involving 572 patients (Davis et al. 1999). Retrospective studies suggest that valproate prevents affective recurrences in bipolar disorder, but only one prospective placebo-controlled study of maintenance with valproate—in which patients were randomized to lithium monotherapy, divalproex monotherapy, or placebo—has been conducted (Solomon et al. 1995). Verapamil and nimodipine have had mood-stabilizing effects in small numbers of cases of bipolar mood disorder, in studies with varying degrees of placebo control. As noted in "Antipsychotic Drugs" (see Chapter 4), clozapine seems more consistently effective as a mood stabilizer than other atypical antipsychotic medications.

The progression in bipolar mood disorders to increased complexity with each recurrence often necessitates combining mood-stabilizing medications when bipolar disorder has been present for a longer period and when it is characterized by rapid cycling and mixed states. Antipsychotic drugs may be necessary adjuncts in maintenance therapy of psychotic bipolar disorder, although as noted in "Bipolar Depression," antipsychotics may increase depressive recurrences in some cases, and atypical antipsychotics can have unpredictable results. ECT is an effective maintenance therapy for bipolar disorder as well as for unipolar depression. However, ECT and lithium have neurotoxic interactions, and anticonvulsants may interfere with the therapeutic effect of ECT. Because it has some anticonvulsant properties, nimodipine could also counteract the therapeutic effect of ECT, but this does not appear to be a problem in actual clinical practice. Therefore, when ECT is used as maintenance therapy, an attempt should be made to limit the number of concomitant medications. The proper frequency of maintenance treatments is determined by gradually increasing the length of time between treatments until early signs of relapse appear.

The efficacy of antimanic drugs in preventing recurrences has been noted to decrease significantly from the first year to the fifth year of treatment. The evolving physiology of bipolar disorder and its interaction with agents such as antidepressants probably contribute to the increasing rate of recurrence over time. In addition, only one-third of outpatients are estimated to remain compliant (Gershon and Soares 1997). In one study, 64% of patients did not adhere to treatment with mood stabilizers in the month preceding hospitalization for acute mania (Keck et al. 1996). During follow-up, 51% of 140 patients recently hospitalized for bipolar disorder were partially or totally noncompliant with pharmacotherapy (Keck et al. 1997).

There are many reasons patients with bipolar mood disorders stop taking their medications. Like patients with unipolar depression, some patients with bipolar disorder avoid the perception of dependence on other people by refusing to depend on medications. Denial of illness, especially in association with manic or hypomanic symptoms, is a common cause of noncompliance. Perhaps even more important is the tendency of some patients to discontinue medications with the expectation that their moods will deteriorate. Feeling that nothing they have done has predictably stabilized their moods, they gain the illusion of control by at least being able to make themselves worse. Patients who have felt well for a significant length of time may have realistic questions about whether they still need active treatment or whether their "thymostats" have reset themselves. The risk of teratogenesis leads many women to discontinue lithium and anticonvulsants in anticipation of pregnancy.

More than 50% of patients experience an affective episode within 6 months of discontinuing lithium therapy, but the risk of recurrence is almost five times as great among patients who discontinue lithium therapy rapidly (median time in remission, 4 months) than among those who taper the dose of the drug over several months (median time in remission, 20 months) (Baldessarini et al. 1996). There is no reason to expect different results with discontinuation of other thymoleptics. Gradual discontinuation of mood stabilizers carries a lower risk of rebound, but relapse is common, especially in patients with highly recurrent illnesses.

Withdrawal of an effective mood stabilizer may also result in refractoriness to treatment with that medication when it is reintroduced. Discontinuation-induced refractoriness may be the result of changes in gene induction and intracellular signaling that arise in an attempt to override medication effects that drive the synapse out of its "default" state. These compensatory changes are overridden by the medication as long as use of it is continued, but they rebound when the medication is withdrawn. Because it is not possible to determine when refractoriness may develop, it is usually recommended that patients continue indefinitely whatever regimen has been effective. If an effective mood stabilizer is to be withdrawn, this should be done very gradually. Dose reductions might be made no more frequently than once a month. This approach reduces the risk of withdrawal and, more importantly, the risk of rebound symptoms. Mood stabilizers that have been prescribed only for a brief period can be withdrawn more rapidly.

Psychotherapy has not been shown to reduce recurrence rates in bipolar disorder, unlike in unipolar depression. This does not mean, however, that psychotherapy is not an important component of maintenance treatment in bipolar disorder. One obvious goal of any form of maintenance psychotherapy is to improve medication compliance. Another is to monitor for early symptoms of recurrence. Interpersonal and social rhythm therapy has been shown to stabilize circadian rhythms, and preliminary evidence suggests that it could enhance the prophylactic effect of mood-stabilizing medications (Frank et al. 1997). If formal interpersonal therapy and logs of circadian cues are not used, the physician can still facilitate mood stabilization, by helping the patient keep regular hours (especially for going to sleep and waking up) and resolving interpersonal and family distress, including unrealistic expectations and high levels of expressed emotion.

Although use for this indication has not been formally studied, expressive psychotherapy can be helpful for addressing the effect of a chronically unstable mood on the patient's personality and outlook. For example, mood lability makes some patients feel like unpredictable, undependable people who cannot get along with anyone; these patients feel that way especially when overstimulated and angry in close relationships. This negative self-concept is enhanced by repeatedly unsatisfactory relationships that make patients want to reject others before they themselves are rejected. Patients who avoid dysphoric overstimulation by becoming withdrawn or reclusive may lose confidence in their social skills. Patients who do not know when their moods will fluctuate next may engage in activities that provoke either depression or hypomania, so that they maintain the illusion of control over a part of themselves that otherwise feels unpredictable and uncontrollable. Understanding these traits as being organized around an unstable mood rather than as personality flaws may help the patient to gain more control over them.

Problems in Maintenance Treatment

Even though there is mounting evidence of the need for indefinite continuation of mood-stabilizing therapies in bipolar disorder, many patients want to withdraw medications after one or more bipolar affective episodes. Many patients find it very difficult to tolerate the gradual changes in regimen that are necessary to maximize long-term mood stability. Patients who are impatient or irritable anyway tend to give up on medications that do not have immediate results, especially if the patients feel depressed. The decision to discontinue treatment is almost inevitable in adolescent patients, who are especially sensitive to the stigma of having to take medications and having something wrong with them. In addition to issues such as not wanting to be ill, many of these patients understandably are not convinced that they require chronic treatment once they feel well, or they are unwilling to submit to the inconvenience and potential adverse effects of maintenance therapy when they might not have another spontaneous episode for many years.

When a patient with a bipolar mood disorder who understands the risks prefers to discontinue treatment, an attempt should be made to withdraw medications as gradually as possible—preferably over at least 3–6 months. If the patient is taking multiple medications, they should be withdrawn one at a time. By staying in touch with the patient and the family, the clinician will be able to help the patient identify subtle signs of early relapse and recurrence and convince him or her to increase the dose gradually or restart treatment with the medication if it has been completely withdrawn. However, it is not uncommon for patients to experience several recurrences before they agree that maintenance treatment is a good idea, at which point the illness may be more difficult to treat.

Many women who are compliant with maintenance treatment prefer to withdraw mood-stabilizing medications in anticipation of pregnancy and breast-feeding. This can sometimes be achieved through gradual withdrawal of treatment before pregnancy begins, because bipolar disorder sometimes goes into remission during pregnancy. Lithium and anticonvulsants can be teratogenic, whereas verapamil and antipsychotic drugs seem less risky. ECT appears to be safe during pregnancy; the very brief exposure to short-acting barbiturates is relatively benign. It is commonly recommended that nursing mothers not take lithium, because a few cases of lithium toxicity have been reported in nursing infants. However, the actual lithium dose is usually very low, and the level is often undetectable; as is true of antidepressants, the patient can minimize the dose to the infant by nursing before taking an evening dose of lithium and by using immediate-release preparations so that peak blood levels after dosing will not be as prolonged. In view of the increased risk of bipolar disorder in postpartum depression and the very substantial likelihood that postpartum psychosis is caused by bipolar disorder, mood stabilizers should be considered seriously in these conditions even if such medications were not used previously.

■ ANTIMANIC DRUGS IN CHILDREN AND ADOLESCENTS

Lithium has not consistently been found to be effective in mania or bipolar depression in younger patients (Kafantaris 1995). It is possible that higher rates of spontaneous improvement, a greater influence of psychosocial factors, and a high rate of response to placebo contribute to the apparent reduced rate of responsiveness to lithium in juvenile bipolar mood disorder, as in unipolar depression. It is also possible that this population requires more frequent dosing or higher serum levels than are necessary for a thymoleptic response in adults. Anticonvulsants have been the subject of open trials (but not placebo-controlled studies) in childhood and adolescent bipolar disorder (Kafantaris 1995). The results of these trials demonstrate that divalproex and carbamazepine are well tolerated and possibly effective. However, carbamazepine sometimes makes children and adolescents more irritable. Verapamil, which is used to treat juvenile cardiac disease, has been used successfully in a few cases of adolescent mania (Kastner and Friedman 1992). Case series and clinical experience indicate that ECT is as effective for treating mania in juvenile patients as it is in adults (Kutcher and Robertson 1995).

All mood-stabilizing medications other than calcium-channel blockers can cause cognitive impairment, which is obviously a concern for students who may have had academic difficulties anyway because of distractibility, racing thoughts, and boredom. If a mood stabilizer eliminates these problems but the patient has cognitive side effects, cognitive dysfunction may respond to the addition of a cholinesterase inhibitor. As discussed in Chapter 4, these medications may have some adjunctive mood-stabilizing properties.

Many adults with severe bipolar disorders can recall having been symptomatic in childhood. However, it is not yet known whether childhood bipolar disorder inevitably continues into adulthood. The course of juvenile bipolar disorder is more chronic than that of adult bipolar disorder (Lewinsohn et al. 1995). In view of data indicating that withdrawal of effective mood stabilizers in children and adolescents is followed by worsening of the illness (Strober et al. 1995), it is probably prudent to continue, through adolescence, to administer medications that do not interfere with academic performance. Until empirical data are accumulated, decisions about the balance between potential positive and negative effects of maintenance medications on affective recurrence and intellectual and personality development are matters of opinion and experience, as is the decision to very slowly institute a trial of no maintenance therapy after adolescence.

■ REFERENCES

American Psychiatric Association: Practice guideline for the treatment of patients with bipolar disorder. Am J Psychiatry 151:1–36, 1994

Baldessarini RJ, Tondo L, Faedda GL, et al: Effects of the rate of discontinuing lithium maintenance treatment in bipolar disorders. J Clin Psychiatry 57:441–448, 1996

Bauer MS, Whybrow PC: Rapid cycling bipolar affective disorder. Arch Gen Psychiatry 47:435–440, 1990

Berman E, Wolpert EA: Intractable manic-depressive psychosis with rapid cycling in an 18-year-old woman successfully treated with electroconvulsive therapy. J Nerv Ment Dis 175:236–239, 1987

Bowden CL, Calabrese JR, McElroy SL, et al: The efficacy of lamotrigine in rapid cycling and non-rapid cycling patients with bipolar disorder. Biol Psychiatry 45:953–958, 1999

Calabrese JR, Bowden CL, Sachs GS, et al: A double-blind placebo-controlled study of lamotrigine monotherapy in outpatients with bipolar I depression. Lamictal 602 Study Group. J Clin Psychiatry 60:79–88, 1999

Calabrese JR, Suppes T, Bowden CL, et al: A double-blind, placebo-controlled, prophylaxis study of lamotrigine in rapid-cycling bipolar disorder. Lamictal 614 Study Group. J Clin Psychiatry 61:841–850, 2000

Calabrese JR, Shelton MD, Bowden CL, et al: Bipolar rapid cycling: focus on depression as its hallmark. J Clin Psychiatry 62 (suppl 14):34–41, 2001

Compton MT, Nemeroff CB: The treatment of bipolar depression. J Clin Psychiatry 61 (suppl 9):57–67, 2000

Davanzo PA, Krah N, Kleiner J, et al: Nimodipine treatment of an adolescent with ultradian cycling bipolar affective illness. J Child Adolesc Psychopharmacol 9:51–61, 1999

Davis JM, Janicak PG, Hogan DM: Mood stabilizers in the prevention of recurrent affective disorders: a meta-analysis. Acta Psychiatr Scand 100:406–417, 1999

Expert Consensus Panel for Bipolar Disorder: Treatment of bipolar disorder. J Clin Psychiatry 57 (suppl 12A):3–88, 1996

Findling RL, Reed MD, Bluner JL: Pharmacological treatment of depression in children and adolescents. Paediatric Drugs 1:161–182, 1999

Frank E, Hlastala S, Ritenour A, et al: Inducing lifestyle regularity in recovering bipolar disorder patients: results from the maintenance therapies in bipolar disorder protocol. Biol Psychiatry 41:1165–1173, 1997

Gershon S, Soares JC: Current therapeutic profile of lithium. Arch Gen Psychiatry 54:16–18, 1997

Gjessing LR: Disturbances of somatic function in catatonia with a periodic course and their compensation. Journal of Mental Science 84:608–621, 1938

Kafantaris V: Treatment of bipolar disorder in children and adolescents. J Am Acad Child Adolesc Psychiatry 34:732–741, 1995

Kallner G, Lindelius R, Petterson U, et al: Mortality in 487 patients with affective disorders attending a lithium clinic or having left it. Pharmacopsychiatry 33:8–13, 2000

Kastner T, Friedman DL: Verapamil and valproic acid treatment of prolonged mania. J Am Acad Child Adolesc Psychiatry 31:271–275, 1992

Keck PE Jr, McElroy SL, Strakowski SM, et al: Factors associated with pharmacologic noncompliance in patients with mania. J Clin Psychiatry 57:292–297, 1996

Keck PE Jr, McElroy SL, Strakowski SM, et al: Compliance with maintenance treatment in bipolar disorder. Psychopharmacol Bull 33:87–91, 1997

Keller MB, Ryan ND, Strober M, et al: Efficacy of paroxetine in the treatment of adolescent major depression: a randomized, controlled trial. J Am Acad Child Adolesc Psychiatry 40 (7):762–772, 2001

Kusumakar V, Yatham LN, Haslam DRS, et al: Treatment of mania, mixed state, and rapid cycling. Can J Psychiatry 42 (suppl 2):79S–86S, 1997

Kusumi I, Ohmori T, Kohsaka M, et al: Chronobiological approach for treatment-resistant rapid cycling affective disorders. Biol Psychiatry 37: 553–559, 1995

Kutcher S, Robertson HA: Electroconvulsive therapy in treatment-resistant bipolar youth. J Child Adolesc Psychopharmacol 5:167–175, 1995

Lewinsohn PM, Klein DN, Seeley JR: Bipolar disorders in a community sample of older adolescents: prevalence, phenomenology, comorbidity, and course. J Am Acad Child Adolesc Psychiatry 34:454–463, 1995

Loo H, Brochier T: Long-term treatment with antidepressive drugs. Ann Med Psychol (Paris) 153:190–196, 1995

McDaniel JS, Musselman DL, Porter MR, et al: Depression in patients with cancer: diagnosis, biology, and treatment. Arch Gen Psychiatry 52 (2):89–99, 1995

McElroy SL, Keck PE Jr, Pope HG Jr, et al: Clinical and research implications of the diagnosis of dysphoric or mixed mania or hypomania. Am J Psychiatry 149:1633–1644, 1992

Moller H-J, Grunze H: Have some guidelines for the treatment of acute bipolar depression gone too far in the restriction of antidepressants? Eur Arch Psychiatry Clin Neurosci 250:57–68, 2000

Mosolov SN, Moshchevitin SL: Use of electroconvulsive therapy for breaking the continuous course of drug-resistant affective and schizoaffective psychoses. Zhurnal Nevropatologii i Psikhiatrii Imeni S.S. Korsakova 90:121–125, 1990

Nolen WA, Bloemkolk D: Treatment of bipolar depression: a review of the literature and a suggestion for an algorithm. Neuropsychobiology 42 (suppl 1):11–17, 2000

Okuma T: Effects of carbamazepine and lithium on affective disorders. Neuropsychobiology 27:138–145, 1993

Pazzaglia PJ, Post RM, Ketter TA, et al: Nimodipine monotherapy and carbamazepine augmentation in patients with refractory recurrent affective illness. J Clin Psychopharmacol 18:404–413, 1998

Post RM: Approaches to treatment-resistant bipolar affectively ill patients. Clin Neuropharmacol 11:93–104, 1988

Post RM, Roy-Byrne PP, Uhde TW: Graphic representation of the life course of illness in patients with affective disorder. Am J Psychiatry 145 (7):844–848, 1988

Post RM, Frye MA, Denicoff KD, et al: Emerging trends in the treatment of rapid cycling bipolar disorder: a selected review. Bipolar Disord 2:305–315, 2000

Reynolds CF 3rd, Kupfer DJ, Thase ME, et al: Sleep, gender, and depression: an analysis of gender effects on the electroencephalographic sleep of 302 depressed outpatients. Biol Psychiatry 28 (8):673–684, 1990

Roy-Byrne P, Post RM, Uhde TW, et al: The longitudinal course of recurrent affective illness: life chart data from research patients at the NIMH. Acta Psychiatr Scand Suppl 317:1–34, 1985

Sachs GS, Printz DJ, Kahn DA, et al: The Expert Consensus Guideline Series: medication treatment of bipolar disorder 2000. Postgrad Med (Spec No):1–104, 2000

Solomon DA, Bauer MS: Continuation and maintenance pharmacotherapy for unipolar and bipolar mood disorders. Psychiatr Clin North Am 16:515–540, 1993

Solomon DA, Keitner GI, Miller IW, et al: Course of illness and maintenance treatments for patients with bipolar disorder. J Clin Psychiatry 56:5–13, 1995

Stancer HC, Persad E: Treatment of intractable rapid-cycling manic-depressive disorder with levothyroxine: clinical observations. Arch Gen Psychiatry 39:311–312, 1982

Strober M, Lackner SS, Freeman R, et al: Recovery and relapse in adolescents with bipolar affective illness: a five-year naturalistic, prospective follow-up. J Am Acad Child Adolesc Psychiatry 34:724–731, 1995

Thase ME, Sachs GS: Bipolar depression: pharmacotherapy and related therapeutic strategies. Biol Psychiatry 48:558–572, 2000

Tohen M, Jacobs TG, Grundy SL, et al: Efficacy of olanzapine in acute bipolar mania: a double-blind, placebo-controlled study. The Olanzapine HGGW Study Group. Arch Gen Psychiatry 57:841–849, 2000

Walden J, Schaerer L, Schloesser S, et al: An open longitudinal study of patients with bipolar rapid cycling treated with lithium or lamotrigine for mood stabilization. Bipolar Disord 2:336–339, 2000

Wolpert EA, Berman V, Bernstein M: Efficacy of electroconvulsive therapy in continuous rapid cycling bipolar disorder. Psychiatric Annals 29:679–683, 1999

Zarate CA Jr, Tohen M, Baldessarini RJ: Clozapine in severe mood disorders. J Clin Psychiatry 56:411–417, 1995

Zornberg GL, Pope HG Jr: Treatment of depression in bipolar disorder: new directions for research. J Clin Psychopharmacol 13:397–408, 1993

AFTERWORD

Mood disorders not only are among the most common medical disorders but also are the most complex. A large body of evidence points increasingly to the fact that it is easier to treat early than later episodes of any mood disorder. Complete treatment of early episodes and continuation of effective therapy reduce the risk of later, more refractory episodes. Unfortunately, denial, reluctance to acknowledge a need for help (because being helped feels like a sign of weakness), pressure from family members who may have mood disorders themselves, and acceptance of a good but incomplete remission make it difficult for people in the early stages of a mood disorder to recognize the seriousness of the illness, let alone obtain treatment. Managed care organizations can support patient denial both by discouraging careful maintenance therapy once acute symptoms seem to have gone away and by failing to recognize psychosocial dysfunction as evidence of incomplete remission.

Public education has reduced the stigma of seeking treatment for mood disorders to some extent, but efforts to educate primary care physicians, whom patients with mood disorders are more likely to visit before mental health professionals, have not been successful in increasing rates of recognition, effective treatment, and, when necessary, referral for specialty care. Research into strategies for approaching mood disorders in primary care practice is therefore as important as research into new treatment technologies.

INDEX

*Page numbers printed in **boldface** type refer to tables or figures.*